MW00386550

AYURVEDA

—

THE POWER TO HEAL

PAUL DUGLISS, M.D.

Nicole,

Wishing You Perfect Health

Paul Dugliss

No part of this book is to be taken as a substitute for medical advice. Consult your health-care provider before making or implementing any changes based on this book.

Copyright © 2007, MCD Century Publications. All rights reserved. No part of this book may be reproduced by any means without the written permission of the publisher.

Cover Design: Ko Wicke, Proglyphics, Royal Oak, MI.
Cover Photos:
> Sun (Background) — Sergey Galushko
> Massage — Niderlander (dreamstime.com)
> Ayurvedic Food and Rudraksha Fruit — Tracy Briney

TABLE OF CONTENTS

Dedicated to my patients.

ACKNOWLEDGEMENTS

I would like to thank all those who have made my life in medicine possible, particularly David McClanahan, Philip Conran, Clinton Greenstone, D. Edwards Smith, Carol Lubetkin, and Maharishi Mahesh Yogi. I would especially like to honor my parents who valued education and inspired and supported me in switching to a career in medicine. Special thanks to Heather Ashare who contributed significantly to the manuscript and provided valuable advice and editing during the production of the manuscript. Also thanks to Michelle Westerdale and Kathleen Chirdon for their editing expertise.

Preface:

A Blessed Life

You hold in your hands a book that is the result of a most blessed life. Through it you will become part of a quiet revolution in health care. I write these words with a profound awareness of what a blessed life I have lived. I have seen incurable diseases cured, the permanently crippled walk, and the infertile give birth. I have seen patients hobble into a clinic with debilitating back pain and walk out pain-free. Through these amazing experiences, I have seen the great potential ancient medicines hold for healing and transforming the lives of people everywhere.

The profession of a physician has not been without its tragedies. I have seen more people die in a few short years of training than most will ever see in several lifetimes. I have seen people cut down in the prime of their lives by cancer, leaving young children and successful careers behind. I have seen men in their early 40s die of heart attacks, and I have seen a 3 year-old die as a result of complications of a tonsillectomy. Having experienced such tragedies, I now hold in my mind the blessing of how precious and delicate life is. It has also steeled my will to do everything in my power to prevent such tragedies from ever occurring and to finding less invasive ways of healing.

Having lived within two cultures — within the modern medical system and the alternative medical world — I have been given the fortune of a unique, firsthand perspective on the problems confronting health care and the solutions that are being overlooked. When I read about the numbers of people injured by medical errors, for me, these statistics are more than numbers. I remember faces and names, friends and colleagues, patients and families who have suffered from these mistakes. When we learn about the number of deaths that occur each year from prescription drugs, I am once again reminded that each of these numbers represents a precious human life that could have been spared.

Year after year, what becomes clearer to me is that these tragedies can be avoided. I am increasingly convinced that we have not even scratched the surface of the potential that the ancient systems of medicine hold for modern life. With the great blessings I have had, I can no longer simply focus on my own private practice integrating modern and ancient medicines. The time has come for the miracles I have witnessed to be commonplace. The time has come for the tragedies to cease. The time has come for a transformation in the practice of medicine.

When David Eisenberg showed in his 1993 *New England Journal of Medicine* article that there are more visits to alternative medicine practitioners than to primary care physicians, it was a wake-up call for the medical profession. We, the people, create the medical system by our passive or active use and acceptance of it. And we are creating an alternative system of medicine through our interest, demand

and practice of ancient medicines such as Ayurveda. With our energy and will directed toward a more enlightened approach to medicine, we cannot fail in transforming medicine. No other approach to medicine is so comprehensive and readily understandable as Ayurveda.

Ayurveda recognizes that we cannot be healthy in isolation. As long as a large proportion of society is ill, we will all be ill. The reality of human existence is that we do not live in isolation. Those with an enlightened perspective know that all life is interrelated. As long as illness exists in the world, none of us can be truly healthy. If we wish to be healthy, if we wish our families to be healthy, our only choice is to create something better. Rather than reinventing what has already been given to us, we are truly fortunate to have the ancient secrets of Ayurveda revealed to us in this modern age.

What you hold in your hands is an introduction to this marvelous system of health and longevity. By learning about your power to heal through Ayurveda, you are participating in one of the most important transformations in history — the transformation of modern medicine. Never before has there been a time when the hidden secrets of health and longevity have been made so widely available. Never before have the advances of one group of people been so instantaneously visible and available to the whole world through modern communications technology. Never before has there been such an opportunity for change and transformation.

The time has come to end the tragedies of modern medicine. The time has come to create real health. The time has come for us to take our health into our own hands and to learn a more enlightened medicine — the natural medicine known as Ayurveda. The time has come for you to fulfill the potential you hold for making perfect health a reality. My hope is that the book you hold in your hands will be the key to a marvelous transformation for yourself and the world. You are the future of medicine.

It is indeed a blessed time and a blessed life.

Paul Dugliss, M.D.

1

THE FABRIC OF THE HEALING PROCESS

This book is about you. It is about your power to heal. It is about the source of this power within you and how to contact it and maximize it. It is about the rediscovery of a whole system of health that can understand and guide the process of healing anything from an emotional hurt to a cut finger to a chronic disease. It is about how we heal. And it is about the blocks to healing and how to eliminate them.

The power to heal is not limited to doctors or nurses or health-care workers. It is a huge, almost unlimited power, as big as nature itself. And still it remains subtle, hidden, and misunderstood. It remains outside the field of normal study. Experts in health abound, but where does one go to study healing? The process is elusive at best, esoteric at worst. Its presence, though, is unmistakable. Consider my patient Susan.

Susan's Story

At 28 years of age, Susan was an electrical engineer for a Detroit automaker. She almost married three years prior while involved with a man she met at work. After they split, she became depressed but continued working. Her depression lifted when she met Sam, a resident in Pediatrics at the University of Michigan. They had been dating for almost two years when she noticed some pressure in her chest. She mentioned this to Sam, who passed it off as insignificant and most likely related to heartburn or reflux. "You are too young to be having a heart attack. It is nothing to worry about." She continued working but had intermittent periods of intense chest pressure.

One day while she was walking up the stairs, a crushing sensation took her breath away. She felt like she might pass out. Alarmed, she rushed to the hospital emergency room. After having multiple vials of blood extracted from her arm, an electrocardiogram (EKG), and a chest x-ray, the emergency room physician came in to assure her that it was not a heart attack.

"Your EKG is normal, and there was no evidence of any damage to the heart in the blood tests we did."

"Thank goodness," said Susan.

"However, we need to send you for a CT scan of the chest," said the ER doctor. "There is a shadow over this area of the heart that we can't decipher, and a CT will help us to know if it is related to your symptoms."

"What does 'a shadow' mean?" asked Susan.

"We don't know. It may be just an artifact. That's why we need the CT," said the doctor.

Several hours passed while Susan waited her turn in the scanner and then awaited the results. For her it seemed like an eternity, but at least she felt like her chest pressure was lessening, and she was getting help. Finally, the curtain surrounding her gurney was pulled aside, and three white-coated individuals appeared.

"Susan, I am Dr. Woolscroft, and these are my residents, Drs. Adam and Ockner. Your ER physician called us to meet with you because of this finding on your CT scan."

He began to point to a blur of gray in the middle of one of many views of what seemed like photographic negatives.

"You have some sort of mass surrounding the main vessels in your heart. It is not at all clear what kind of mass this could be, and we will need to admit you to the hospital for a couple of days to do some further testing and sort all of this out."

Susan was stunned.

"But I am feeling fine. I just have some tightness in the chest occasionally. Why do I have to stay?"

"Susan, this mass is constricting the blood supply to the heart. That can be dangerous. What we need to do is determine immediately what type of tumor this is and whether it can be operated on. If we sent you home, you might pass out driving on the way," said Dr. Woolscroft.

After he finished explaining the tests that would be undertaken in the next couple of days, Susan was transferred up to the hospital floor. She called her friends whom she had met in a meditation group from Ann Arbor and made arrangements for them to watch her cat and bring her some books.

When they arrived, she had little intention of reading the books she had requested but instead wanted to sit with her friends quietly to meditate together. Once they had finished their 15-minute meditation, Susan asked if they could meet again the following day. Her friends obliged without hesitation.

During the night, Susan's sleep was light and interrupted. She kept thinking that this mass around her heart must have something to do with her emotions, with her *feeling* heart. After her friends came the next morning and meditated with her, Susan decided to finally call Sam.

"Why didn't you call me immediately?" he yelled. "I am coming right over."

"No," said Susan. "I have a lot of tests scheduled, and I need to do some thinking. Come over tonight."

The day passed, and the next day further tests were ordered. A thoracic surgeon was consulted.

"Susan," he said, "I have looked at your MRI. Even if we removed it, we could not excise the entire mass, leaving it free to grow right back. I unfortunately can be of no service to you."

Another day passed with more meetings with more doctors. Finally, Dr. Woolscroft appeared.

"We want you to consider having a stent put in to keep the blood flow open. Then you should begin radiation therapy. Since surgery is out of the question, radiation is the only hope for this type of tumor. You can go home day after tomorrow after the stent is put in."

"We'll see," replied Susan. "I am not sure yet that I want that hardware in me. I was really doing fine. I just had some chest pressure."

The doctors continued trying to convince her. She agreed to think about it overnight. That evening she called Sam into her room.

"Sam, I know this is the worst time to being doing this. I have done a lot of thinking these last few days. I love you. I really do. But you have such a dominating personality. I think that is what may have attracted me to you in the first place. I have meditated a lot and thought a lot, and I know in my heart that I must end this relationship if I am to survive. I know that this is not fair to you and that you will be agonizing about me and my health. But I just know that I have to let go of you now.

Susan ended the relationship and went home the next day without the stent. She was scheduled to meet with the radiation oncologist in 12 days. She spent a lot of time with friends. She missed Sam but had made up her mind. She was feeling less chest pressure but still was taking it easy.

In order to fit the radiation ports to her body and her tumor, she had to undergo another MRI scan on the day she was to meet with the radiation oncologist. After waiting for two hours following the MRI, she was ushered into a room with several white-coated individuals. She recognized Dr. Davis, the radiation oncologist she had met while still in the hospital.

"Susan," he said, shaking his head. "I don't know how to explain this to you. I have gone over your initial MRI taken at the time you went into the hospital. I have checked and double-checked your previous results and the MRI today. I have had a radiologist and another oncologist go over these."

"What is the problem, Dr. Davis?" asked Susan.

"Well," he said, "There is no tumor on the MRI we did today. It is gone. Completely gone. I don't understand it. But it is no mistake."

"I understand it," said Susan. "There *was* something constricting my heart... and it is no longer there."

A Search to Understand Healing

Susan's is a story of dramatic healing. It is a story of the amazing potential we all have to heal the body. Why does it happen so rarely? Why can't every cancer patient heal this way, without surgery or chemotherapy? Yet how do we harness this possibility, and who understands the process for making this happen reliably?

Susan's story sets expectations extremely high. For many, this type of healing simply does not occur. They are drawn into a belief that the mind can heal anything and feel defeated when they can't remain optimistic in the face of a serious disease like cancer.

While Susan's story points out the fact that we have an almost unlimited healing potential, it does not explain *how* healing happens and why it happened to her and for so few others. Without a deep understanding of the nature of the mind, there is little hope that this type of healing can be consistently replicated. But as this knowledge is gained, the full potential comes within our grasp.

How does healing occur, and what is the role of consciousness, mind and emotions in this process?

My search to answer these questions began more than 20 years ago. At that time I was drawn to the knowledge of the East. It seemed an incredible untapped source, given the modern fixation on biochemical science. I came to this conclusion later, after pursuing my interest in curing some minor problems of my own with herbs.

The year was 1984, and I had from my adolescent years developed an interest in psychology and had pursued a master's degree in clinical and counseling psychology. While working as a psychologist in a community hospital psychiatric ward, I began studying Chinese medicine. If at that point you had mentioned I would one day become a physician, I would have laughed at such a preposterous notion despite my fascination with Chinese medicine.

It was through this study that I was introduced to Dr. Wen-wie Xie, a physician from Beijing, China. He was in his last year of a fellowship, doing research at Case Western Reserve University and the Cleveland Clinic. Dr. Xie told me he wanted to give back some of his knowledge to the United States, a country from which he had learned so much. He asked me to help organize a study group for traditional Chinese medicine. I was very excited to do this. Our group met every week at my house, and we began importing herbs from China to study.

Dr. Xie gave me the privilege of sitting in on his consultations and he encouraged me in my studies. Through him I began the study of pulse diagnosis. One day Dr. Xie mentioned that he had been working with a researcher named

E. Pedigo to develop a new form of Transcutaneous Electrical Nerve Stimulation, or TENS.

In 1985, I was invited to Mr. Pedigo's pain clinic near Cleveland, Ohio, to witness this new medical therapy.

"What is unique about the machine I have developed is that it can detect the exact location of the acupuncture meridians and indicate to the therapist the correct placement of the electrodes," Mr. Pedigo said, pointing to several acupuncture charts on his walls.

He then used the machine to locate one of his own meridians. The meter on the machine jumped when the channel was located. As interesting as this was, I was not prepared for what I witnessed next.

After a short introduction, Mr. Pedigo brought in a severely disabled patient who agreed to let me watch his first treatment. The patient had been paralyzed for six years from the waist down due to a terrible accident. After several minutes of treatment, Mr. Pedigo asked the patient to move his right toe.

"Listen, Doc, I can't move nothing," he snapped.

Mr. Pedigo adjusted the equipment and told him to try again. This time he was able to move the toe. I was stunned and perplexed as I sat there wondering how this occurred. And I was, at the same time, deeply inspired to have witnessed firsthand this miracle.

Six months later, this patient could walk with the assistance of a walker and cane. As an eager and curious 29-year-old, I was immediately pulled into a quest to know as much as I could about the wisdom ancient systems of medicine have for healing these stubborn and severe problems.

Since that time I have witnessed many such miracles — incurable diseases cured, sanity regained, nicotine addicts forgetting to smoke, and crippling back pain alleviated. These are just a few examples of the great power that ancient medicines hold for healing and transforming people everywhere. But it was not until I attended medical school and became an internist that I finally discovered a systematic understanding of healing through the ancient East Indian medicine known as *Ayurveda*.

The word *Ayurveda* comes from two Sanskrit words: "Ayur," meaning life or longevity, and "Veda," meaning knowledge or truth. Ayurveda, then, can be translated as "knowledge of longevity" or the "truth of life." Both meanings convey the profound understanding of the nature of health and healing contained within this system of medicine.

Ayurveda is more than 5,000 years old and is considered the mother of all natural medicines, having given rise to Tibetan medicine and then Chinese medicine, as well as Greek medicine. It is a complete system of medicine, and many are surprised to learn that it contains surgery as one of its subspecialties.

Sushruta was the most famous Ayurvedic surgeon. He lived around 220 BC and designed many of the instruments used in modern surgery. He described more than 60 operations on the eye alone and was able to perform amazing reconstructive surgeries — one of which is still used today in reconstructive surgery and is called the "Indian flap." Sushruta is the Indian referred to in the name of this technique.

However, Sushruta's surgical expertise went far beyond fine motor skill. His phenomenal success was created by a refined understanding of health and healing in Ayurveda. Sushruta understood the flow of energy in the body and which energy flows should not be cut through if healing were to take place normally. He understood health and what creates it. He gave it this definition:

> *He whose* Doshas [physiologic functions] *are in balance, whose appetite is good, whose* Dhatus [tissue layers] *are functioning normally, whose* Malas [body wastes] *are in balance, and whose body, mind and senses remain full of bliss* [24 hours a day]*, is called a healthy person.*

This is a positive definition of health, not just "an absence of disease."

Sushruta described the subtle signs and flows that indicate the balanced functioning of the *Doshas*, how to assess the tissue layers, and what clues the qualities of wastes give in determining the healthy recreation of tissue. Most importantly, though, he emphasized the connection between mind and body. Health of the body is an expression of bliss of the mind and the transformations that it guides. The truly healthy person experiences bliss in mind, bliss through the senses, and bliss in the body.

It may seem ludicrous or fanciful for a surgeon to be considering bliss in health. We know that Sushruta must have had incredible insight into the workings of the human frame in order to be able to perform the incredible operations he detailed and taught to his students. His astute insight requires that we as individuals and health professionals dramatically shift our way of thinking about the body and its capacity to heal.

What is Health?

If we are to utilize our potential to heal, we must first understand health. Sushruta gives us the signs and clues of health, but what is it actually? The word "heal" comes from Old English *heilen* or *hal*, which means to make whole (as in "hale and hardy"). Health, then, is wholeness. If health comes from the root "wholeness," where is this wholeness found? What are we no longer a part of, or what are we cut off from, when we are no longer "whole" or healthy? And what do we have to reconnect to in order to become whole again?

To answer these questions we must understand the source of our awareness and of our liveliness. The term "holistic health" is not simply about nonphysical therapies. It is about understanding the source of healing that brings about the relief of suffering, whether the modality is massage therapy, acupuncture, herb therapy, or psychotherapy. It is the source of life, of awareness, out of which healing originates. It is the source of life energy that is contacted in the process.

Understanding the nature of the source of life and of health, and understanding the modifications of the vibrations of this underlying field of life is the forte of Ayurvedic medicine. It describes how to reconnect with wholeness, with one's essential nature, and with the source of life. In describing to us how to create health, it is simply describing what our true nature is. It should not be misconstrued that Ayurveda is the source of truth. It is a science that describes the source of truth, as do many sciences and systems. Ayurveda gives us glances and glimpses into the extraordinary workings of the human being.

Ayurveda understands that healing is natural. It is our nature to become whole again. Just as when you cut your finger, you don't have to think to heal the wound. It takes place naturally, continuously, and effortlessly. Ayurveda presupposes that all healing is encoded in the framework of our bodies, minds, and spirits.

The body's natural tendency to heal itself is continuously expressed on the physical level. Each day old cells are replaced flawlessly. Each day the immune system disposes of debris, viruses, and bacteria and keeps the integrity of the body from being compromised by outside influences. Each day the cells undergo restructuring and repair.

Healing and the tendency to make whole again is expressed on every level of the human being. On the emotional level is the universal quality of love. Love seeks to unite, ignoring differences. It accepts and joins together. On the spiritual level is the tendency to want to "go with God," to be at one with the power that underlies creation. Every aspect of our being is preprogrammed to create wholeness.

Healing is organized and intelligent, yet it does not require our will. We don't think about our immune system or will it to work. It flows and works by itself. Healing, technically, is complex. When you cut your finger, an amazingly complex series of automatic healing occurs. Proteins are restructured, a clotting factor is activated, and collagen is formed to recreate the skin structure. Just the clotting cascade alone takes pages to describe, with 13 clotting factors having been characterized. Whole chapters exist in medical textbooks on the clotting factors and what goes wrong when one is deficient. Yet, all of this intelligent functioning takes place without our active awareness or participation.

Healing is Allowed

Healing is allowed, not willed. Conscious effort can be made to foster the healing process, but ultimately healing occurs through harmony, not force. An example of this fact is found in Jack Schwarz. In the late 1960s and early 1970s the Menninger Foundation attempted to research various yogis and mystics. Jack was one of these. The Menninger Foundation was aware of the growing research of biofeedback and wanted to understand the limits of human potential to control and influence the physical body. Jack Schwarz was studied for many different abilities, but the most impressive of which was his ability to take a knitting needle and pass it through his biceps, remove it, and control the bleeding. In reviewing the films of this demonstration, it was observed that his skin would actually start to show spontaneous healing at the site of the wound. The researchers asked how he was able to do this and how he could control the bleeding and heal the wound so quickly.

"I don't control the bleeding. I don't control the body," he said. "I ask the body if it will allow me to pass the needle through the arm."

Jack Schwarz demonstrated a key to the process of healing — it is allowed, not controlled. I have had several patients describe this phenomenon with the process of meditation. In letting go, healing takes place without focus on the problem area. Wounds are healed, migraines cured, depression banished, all seemingly without purposefully making the healing happen.

We cannot understand this process solely through the study of biochemistry. It is not a thought system that lends itself to explain and comprehend how such healing can occur. We are much more than just physical beings. The sum of our parts is much greater than just parts connected together. Physical theories of the human being can only go so far, as they often leave off the most important part of us: that part which makes us human.

To understand this process of healing, we must understand a different view of the human being and how it functions, one that goes far beyond the physical model. With this new perspective, we will be able to begin the journey to utilizing our full potential for healing and health.

2

THE SOURCE OF HEALING

The Sign is Not the Place

The model of the human being is just that, a model. No concept, scheme, or construct can ever describe the entire complexity of the human being and its physiology. This is like the story of the young boy who asked his uncle what the moon was. The uncle pointed to the moon, and the boy thought for the longest time the moon was a pointed finger.

What follows is a model for the reality that the body is more than a physical system. It is also an energetic system. That being said, the body is not just energy. We are more complex than that. This model is not reality. It is a way to understand reality and how we heal.

We are Nonmaterial Beings

This model is one that makes use of some scientific facts to point to the big picture. In the grand scheme of any given life, the body is really a fleeting event. If you have the assumption that you *are* your body, that your cells have somehow gotten together and created a mind, then you have to know you were not here a year ago. Consider these facts:

- 98 percent of the molecules that make up the body are replaced in one year's time.

- The lining of the stomach replaces itself in five days. Liver cells are constantly being destroyed and replaced. Cut off a lobe of the liver, and it can replace itself in two months.

- Even the most solid part of us, our skeletal system, gets replaced continuously. Bone is constantly being reabsorbed and rebuilt. Osteoporosis is then the end result when there is an imbalance within this regeneration process.

Given these facts, the person you saw in the mirror this morning was not there a year ago. The body has been almost entirely replaced. Even brain cells, once thought not to regenerate, are constantly replacing their internal structure, if not creating new dendrites and losing old ones. The body is impermanent, yet we still persist. The only logical conclusion is that we are not just our physical bodies.

Another way to reach this understanding is to look at human memory. The human brain contains within it approximately 100 billion neurons. Yet despite this enormously vast number, we know these cells are highly organized in terms of their function. The cells at the back of the brain, for instance, relate to visual functions and to the processes responsible for sight, while large areas of the brain relate to movement and balance. However, even if the entire brain were utilized just for memory, it would still not be sufficient to store all the data that an average human can maintain and access.

Consider movies as an example. We have learned how to digitize movies and place the images in a sophisticated and compact manner on a CD-ROM disc called a DVD. Including sound, this process requires, with the best compression techniques, at least 500 megabytes of storage on the disc. Five hundred megabytes are 500 million bytes of information.

If the brain were to use this very elaborate compression system, it would still require a half billion brain cells in order to store the memory of an entire movie. Even utilizing a fourth of all the brain cells for memory storage, the most any human being could possibly store in their brains would be around 50 movies — and this would not allow for storage of any other memories or information, auditory or visual.

If memories were stored in brain cells, then when you reached the point of seeing more than 50 movies, there would be no storage left, and you would start losing older information, like your name and what your parents looked like. Obviously the brain does not lose information in this manner. It does not get full and start writing new memories on top of old ones.

Most people don't recall all the scenes of a movie. However, research has shown when prompted, they can retrieve the memory. For example, many people know the movie *Titanic* with Kate Winslet and Leonardo DiCaprio. Since the movie was popular many years ago, most will not be able to recall much about the film, but *if prompted*, they will be able to recall when Leonardo DiCaprio takes Kate Winslet up to the bow of the boat without her being able to see and then asks her to open her eyes. Most people who saw the movie will recall the scene, *when prompted*. If one can be prompted to recall the memory, then it must therefore exist.

The brain can hold hundreds of movies, hundreds of books, thousands of words, multiple languages, images, thoughts, feelings, and memories. Even with the advantage of the most sophisticated compression algorithms, there are just too few cells in the brain to store all the information. So where is it stored?

The only logical conclusion is that it is not stored in the brain. But if not in the brain, then where? Consider the possibility that the information does not reside in the brain but in a field of energy and intelligence that the brain can access.

The Underlying Field

The ever-changing nature of the body and the concept of the brain as being insufficient to contain all our memories gives rise to a fundamental shift in our thinking about who we are. The brain is not a complex computer that stores and creates thoughts. Logically, this is not possible. The brain functions, instead, to amplify signals from an underlying field. The brain is like an amplifier in your radio. You select a certain station to tune into — for instance, a certain thought — and this is amplified or brought to awareness. Because we know the brain can perceive a single photon or a single quantum of green light, we know the brain can operate on the quantum mechanical level.

This means the human being is not essentially a physical being. Everyone knows that a corpse, while still possessing all the parts of a living body, is not the same as a live human being. Even if we cause the dead body's lungs to move and stimulate its heart to beat with drugs, it is different from a living being who is on a respirator. So how do we objectively know the difference?

One of the criteria that helps doctors determine if someone on a respirator is dead is the electrical activity of the brain. A fundamental difference in brainwave activity exists in a living human being, which points out the fact we are essentially energetic beings who utilize energy and information contained in an underlying field. This is a profoundly different view from the modern medical one that focuses on the physical and chemical structure of the body. This model of the human being goes far beyond simple physical events in attempting to explain wholeness, health, and healing.

We know from experiments with frog embryos that biology is affected by surrounding energy fields. If you pass an electromagnetic current perpendicular to the developing spine in a frog embryo, the frog will develop deformities. If you pass the current parallel to the spine, it develops normally. In this manner energy fields surrounding biological systems can guide or hinder the normal physical function.

If we are all just energy in the same field, why do we have the sense of being isolated and separate from other people? If psychics have the unique ability to tap into others' memories, why can't we all?

In order to understand how this phenomenon takes place, imagine a large pool with a wave machine. Over the pool lies a fish net. Suppose the fish net was lined with a special refrigerating device that could instantly freeze the water above the net, while leaving the water below it liquid. Then suppose we place the net a foot above the surface level of the pool so that only the very crests of the tall waves are above the net. The waves then freeze, and we have a set of individual crests, each unique.

Suppose each crest could be animated with a personality and awareness. One crest would look out and see other crests, each different, each individual and separate. Now let's do the same experiment but lower the level of the net. What happens? We end up with each crest having greater depth, more awareness of what is at its base. Eventually, if we lower the level of the net sufficiently into the pool, each of the waves becomes connected to the others through the water from which they arise. The level of the net corresponds with the "level" of awareness of the underlying field.

Suppose an individual wave named Fred is somehow able to become aware of the underlying pool of water and starts to sense some of the smaller flows and vibrations that are affecting the next crest over. Suddenly, Fred is able to get some impressions of what his fellow wave is experiencing. Fred has become a "psychic" wave.

In this manner, we are individual beings, essentially non-material and independent, yet connected, as we are all part of the same pool, the same ocean. What is the water? The water is consciousness. Our consciousness is that which is connected to a sea of consciousness, and that sea contains tremendous energy, information, and intelligence.

The model of the human being described in Ayurvedic medicine is a consciousness model. Consciousness can be thought of in terms of energy, like electricity or light, but it is much more than that. It contains intelligence, organization, and creativity. Consciousness is the creative force that underlies creation.

At the base of the sea of consciousness there are no waves, just stillness. On the surface, waves and vibrations form. Like any vibration, these are composed of different frequencies.

What do these different frequencies represent? Human physiology is essentially designed for the transformation of these various frequencies to create our thoughts, feelings, and the energy that informs our physical being, as well as our awareness of them.

Consciousness is like a white light, and the human being is like a prism. We transform energy and create various colors through various energy centers in the body. Perhaps a more accurate analogy is electricity as it comes from the source, the power plant. At 100,000 volts, the electricity from its source would fry any electrical device in your home.

As the electrical energy travels from the power station to your home and ultimately to an outlet to power your kitchen blender, the energy is down-regulated at various substations as it makes this journey. So the voltage, which began at 100,000 volts from the power plant, becomes just 110 volts by the time it reaches your home.

Like the power plant, consciousness at its source has tremendous power. Unlike electricity, though, it contains the intelligence for the many forms it inhabits. The various aspects of human existence such as the spirit, mind, emotions, or the body are the expressions of the various frequencies of consciousness. Just like a prism and the frequencies of light that form different colors, our entire existence is organized around transforming energy and consciousness into the human experience.

Three Basic Principles

Three important principles are to be derived from this consciousness model:

- Whenever the flow of consciousness, its intelligence and energy are blocked, the potential for disorganization and disease is created.

- Health is recreated when contact is made with the source of consciousness. This reconnection re-establishes wholeness in the individual.

- Consciousness is a creative force. Just as the section of the garden that we water grows, our consciousness enlivens whatever we place our attention on.

The template for the proper unfolding of the physiology and the tissues exists like a blueprint in a person's consciousness. If the construction foreman loses the blueprints of his project and does not possess a backup set of instructions, the construction project is at serious risk of failing.

Health is maintained or interrupted in an analogous manner. It nurtured by the frictionless flow of energy and intelligence that takes place through the transformations of consciousness. It is frictionless because it does not involve will or effort. Optimal health is preprogrammed into the nature of the human being to transform consciousness into matter and ultimately into the human experience.

The various levels of existence — the spiritual, mental, emotional, etheric (the energy level that feeds the physical), and physical — are not simply concepts about separate states of being that exist when we simply ponder them. They are actual fields with different levels of vibrations, just like the levels of the ocean, that function at particular frequencies.

For instance, as an irate supervisor yells, "I am not angry," she has tapped into two different levels of existence. She has part of her consciousness in the level of mental existence by voicing these words, and at the same time, she has part of it in the level of emotional existence, which is characterized by her feelings of anger.

Dysfunction occurs when the levels are not integrated. When we say one thing and feel another, we become fragmented and disconnected as these levels of ourselves are no longer in agreement. Moreover, a whole and healthy life follows not just when the levels of ourselves are in compatible communication with one another but when these levels are in contact with their source of consciousness.

The Flow

Seven consciousness or energy transformers exist in the human physiology, each associated with different vibrations, functions, and psychospiritual issues. Those who have studied yoga know these as *Chakras*. Buddhist thought sometimes refers to them as the seven lotuses. They are described in terms of location, level of vibration of consciousness, psychology, and physiology. On a physical level each relates to one of the endocrine organs in the body.

In Ayurveda they are called *Mahamarmas* or the great *Marmas*. Just like acupuncture points, they are responsible for the transformation of energy and consciousness into subtle flows through the channels or *Srotas* of the body.

The flow of consciousness starts at the *absolute*, where the frequency of vibration is so high, it is immeasurable, hence the name "absolute". It flows into the next levels all the way down until it reaches the physical level. Any blockage in its flow can create problems. Thus, disease can have its origins on different levels — spiritual, mental, emotional, etheric, or physical. Knowing the level on which the blockage is occurring and how to rebalance it is one of the key components of Ayurvedic medicine.

Not every blockage is a psychological issue or a spiritual one. Put a poison in your body, and the problem is not on the psychological level. Positive thinking or resolving blockages to spiritual power cannot solve it.

The unbridled enthusiasm that accompanied the discovery of mind-body medicine led too many people to believe they could heal anything just by changing their minds. Ayurveda recognizes that disease can arise on many levels and that the wise healer addresses the root cause. This means addressing problems on the appropriate level.

The Three Imperatives

This consciousness model gives us three imperatives, which are three keys to health. The first is that reconnecting with the source of health, the power source, is vital to the process of healing.

The second imperative is that the smooth flow of consciousness or energy to the physical level must be maintained for health to be optimal. An obstruction on any level can hamper the flow of intelligence and energy necessary for natural healing. For instance, cancer can sometimes be due to a physical process, like pollution in the water supply, and sometimes it is due to emotional toxicity. Removing the toxins and the blockage before disease arises is considered a high form of prevention.

The third imperative is that we must animate that which is life-giving and life-promoting. It originates in the principle that awareness can give life to anything. Consciousness is creative in its essence and like a garden, whatever area we water grows. In a similar fashion, we must place our awareness on that which is in tune with our higher nature in order to create a more balanced lifestyle. We must attend to that diet and routine that is in tune with our individual nature.

Since we have thus far concentrated on the theoretical concepts of health, we will now turn our focus onto the practical applications from this model, which utilize the knowledge of Ayurveda to optimize health and healing. We will begin by putting the first imperative into practice, which stresses the importance of contacting the source of power, intelligence, energy, and healing.

3

CONTACTING THE SOURCE

Victoria's Secret

Victoria came to my clinic first when she was 33 years old. She was married and had been trying to conceive since she was 28 years of age. Both she and her husband had been thoroughly tested, but nothing conclusive was discovered. She had been to a gynecologist who specialized in infertility and was put on fertility drugs several times, but she was still unable to conceive.

Victoria was a highly successful businesswoman who jogged 3 miles per day and was active in her church. She was the person her brothers and sisters turned to for help. She slept six hours a night on a good night.

Needless to say, when I started her Ayurvedic assessment, it was clear from her pulse and other subtle signs that she was essentially exhausted. I asked her how much she would be willing to change in order to have a child.

"I'll quit my job, stand on my head, do anything that is necessary," she answered. "Besides," she said, "I am considering a job change anyway."

I explained to Victoria that we have only so many sources of energy. Sometimes these sources, like sleep and nutrition, get depleted and are in need of being replenished. This was clearly the case with Victoria. I talked with her about diet and about herbs but emphasized one significant point:

"I don't care if you continue to work, but you must throw away your alarm clock."

"What? But how will I get up in the morning?" she asked.

"You must get to bed sufficiently early to allow your body to take the rest it needs, so that you wake up naturally."

After much discussion it was obvious to Victoria that her body was essentially protecting her by not allowing her to become pregnant when she was so exhausted and drained. She worked out an agreement with her employer to take a month's vacation and began a new program of diet, herbs, and rest.

After the first week of her Ayurvedic program she reported back to my office.

"I have been sleeping almost 13 hours a night. I felt really sluggish the first four days, but I am beginning to feel more awake. I just feel like the days are so short. How will I ever go back to work?" said Victoria.

"This is normal. Sleep debt is like credit card debt. It is constantly tracked. You have to pay it off sooner or later. When you get some of the debt paid off, the payments become less and much easier to make. After you pay off some of the debt, you won't need to sleep so much," I reassured her. "And your body will function that much better."

We reviewed her diet and herb program and made some adjustments. I recommended she start reading about meditation, consider some yoga, and cut back her jogging to 1 mile per day. She said she actually was noticing that she felt a bit better, a bit lighter already and agreed to continue on the program.

After two weeks her sleep decreased to 10 per night. By the third week she was down to 8 hours per night. She was beginning to recognize that she had been fatigued so long she forgot what it was to be well-rested.

We met several times in the next three months. She was able to work part time and could see clearly now how important sleep was to her mood and her sense of well-being. Two months later she became pregnant and was able to give birth to a healthy 8-pound, 2-ounce girl.

A year later at a prevention class I was teaching she introduced herself to the class. "My name is Victoria, and Dr. Dugliss got me pregnant."

To quickly turn the attention away from my reddening face, I asked, "So tell the class, then, what is Victoria's secret?"

Without hesitation she declared, "Sleep. It was the key to regaining my health."

Three Ways of Contacting the Source

When we are ill, the first recommendation of most physicians is to rest. Most of us know to rest when we are ill, not just because we are weak, but because we know it helps. That is why there are "sick days" offered by most employers. Yet few of us know to rest before we are ill.

Modern medicine still does not have a definitive reason for why we need to sleep. The best and most explained theory at this point is that sleep somehow allows the replenishment of certain neurotransmitters and biochemical substances that the body won't produce well when awake.

From the consciousness model, however, sleep is no mystery. It is one of the ways we contact the source of energy and intelligence that makes up our liveliness and our consciousness. Sleep is not just time when we are lazy. It is an indispensable re-energizing process. Brain functioning shifts dramatically as we sleep, allowing the source to be contacted and the rejuvenation process to take place. The dramatic shift in the brainwaves produced during sleep is evidence for this very active and crucial part of our daily routine.

Sleep is not the only time we go beyond the thinking and sensing mind and contact subtler states of consciousness. This sometimes happens spontaneously during our waking day when we have so-called "peak experiences."

The psychologist Abraham Maslow described the experience of certain individuals when they suddenly are thrown into a higher state of functioning during these "peak experiences." Often these occur during performances or athletic events. During these moments, their action becomes effortless, and their mind holds supreme clarity. It is as if one steps outside of the physical boundaries of his or her body as time slows down, and each movement happens automatically without thought. Interviews with those who have experienced this state express an internal sense of silence, peace, and bliss in the midst of dynamic activity.

The challenge with peak experiences is their lack of reproducibility. It is not possible to consistently create this type of transcendence during activity. However, it is possible to reach this altered state of existence during meditation. During a meditative state, the meditator attempts to dissolve the mind of all thoughts by various processes of focused concentration. Although the goals of meditation are varied, it invokes the guidance of a higher power as the individual seeks to turn the mind's attention inward. In viewing meditation this way, it is a highly efficient and consistent way of contacting the source of health, healing, and wholeness.

There are, then, three ways of contacting the source — through peak experiences, sleep, and meditation. Of these, sleep and meditation make up the most reliable and usable of the three ways. Ayurvedic medicine recognizes the importance of this contact and has very specific and practical recommendations for maximizing their effectiveness.

1) Sleep

Our knowledge of sleep and its effects come from researchers studying the lack of it. In this country, sleep deprivation is very costly. More automobile accidents and deaths are caused each year from insufficient rest than from drunk driving. Moreover, it is estimated that billions of dollars each year are lost in productivity due to our inability to meet our sleep requirements.

As mentioned before, every aspect of human life depends on the awareness you bring to it. Awareness is key. Being conscious of what is going on inside and outside of you is essential. The more aware you are of your environment, the more likely you are to make the changes that ensure your safety. The more deliberate attention you apply to your thoughts and feelings, the more you will be able to understand the relationships in your life. And the more we learn about how the foods we eat and the lifestyle we live affect our sense of well-being, the more able we will be to make choices that will allow us to feel and be a certain way.

Awareness is dependent on human physiology. In order to maximize our awareness, we must clear the way for proper physiologic functioning to occur. The body is the tool through which we perceive reality. Our perception of our reality is imprinted by what we have learned to be real and by the physical state of our bodies. For instance, if one takes a kitten and raises it in an environment that has only vertical lines, the cat will not be able to perceive horizontal lines when it is grown. It will trip over large cracks in the cement, as if it were blind. Likewise, if one takes a group of individuals and deprives them of sleep for 72 hours, they will begin to misperceive their surroundings and see things that are not there. They will start to mistake patterns in the carpet for bugs, or pictures in the wallpaper for birds. In essence, they will start to hallucinate. Proper physiological functioning is therefore mandatory for perceiving reality.

Proper rest is needed for optimal physiologic functioning. We have all experienced a dearth of sleep at some point in our lives and are familiar with the negative impact it can have on our mental and physical health.

Sleep occurs in stages characterized by the type or frequency of brainwaves and muscle activity of the sleeper. There are four stages of sleep, the deepest being stage IV, where slow delta waves are produced. REM sleep, an additional stage, follows stage IV.

REM (which stands for rapid eye movement) sleep is characterized by flaccidity in the body's muscles (with the exception of the eye muscles) and by large-amplitude discharges of brainwaves. Most of our vividly recalled dreams take place during REM sleep.

Most of us have experienced the rejuvenating effects of a good night's sleep after a stressful day. In this stage, it has been theorized that stress is being released from the nervous system. Sleep helps to release the impact of the previous day's stress. Since the largest amount of REM sleep occurs toward morning, if you consistently cut out the last hour of sleep, you are repeatedly preventing this stress-releasing process from occurring. But the good news is that if you get enough rest, you will function more optimally and will hopefully be in a better mood as you go about your day.

Good sleep taken at the proper time is a key component of Ayurveda's preventive health guidelines. It is not simply emphasized when one is ill. It allows integration and growth of the nervous system. The deeper the rest, the more profound the integration. One of the most often quoted classics in Ayurvedic medicine comes from a sage physician Charaka who described thousands of years ago what aspects of life are dependent on proper sleep:

Happiness and misery, growth and wasting, strength and weakness, virility and sterility, knowledge and ignorance, life and death all depend upon sleep.[1]

This is no minor list. Every aspect of health and life is dependent on this often-forgotten blessing according to Ayurvedic reasoning. Because the effects are not immediate, people often deceive themselves into thinking that missing sleep has little consequence. The accumulation of poor sleep over time — cutting sleep regularly, staying up later just to catch Leno — negatively affects the body and your health.

In regard to prevention, Charaka also compared nutrition and sleep:

In the matter of keeping up the body, sleep is regarded to be productive of as much happiness as the taking of food.[2]

It should be noted that happiness in Ayurveda is the end result of health or wholeness. Thus happiness is the reward for "keeping up the body." From this perspective, sleep is on a parallel with food in producing ill or good health.

William C. Dement is perhaps the world's most famous sleep researcher. In his book, *The Promise of Sleep*, he confirms Charaka's saying regarding longevity by providing scientific research that sleep and longevity are connected. He cites a massive research study undertaken in the 1950s, when more than 1 million Americans were surveyed about their exercise, nutrition, smoking, sleep, and other health-related habits. The survey was repeated in six years, and all of the respondents who had died in the meantime were identified. Out of all of the lifestyle factors investigated, habitual sleep time had the best correlation with mortality. This so often overlooked aspect of lifestyle was more predictive of mortality than even nutrition.[3]

2) Meditation

As mentioned previously, meditation is the most reliable way of contacting the source of healing that exists within us. Because of its association with relaxation therapies and stress-management programs, its ability to facilitate healing is often overlooked. Meditation is a way to go beyond the thinking mind and contact the more potent inner regions of consciousness. When all aspects of the conscious thinking mind are transcended, it serves as a direct way to contact the source of liveliness and health.

Jane's Story

Jane T. came to my office when I was supervising a medical student interested in alternative therapies. Jane spoke so quietly that the medical student and I could barely understand her. She was severely depressed and cried through much of the interview. She had been under the care of a psychiatrist who tried putting her on numerous medications. She was on two antidepressants and one antipsychotic medication at the time of our first meeting. She could hardly hold her head up. She could not make eye contact. I asked the medical student to leave the interview after a short while, hoping this would make her feel more comfortable. It did not help in the least.

We discussed the Ayurvedic approach to treating depression, and I emphasized the role of meditation as part of this approach. We also talked about her daily routine of medications. I suggested we hold off on herbal therapy until I could research interactions between her antipsychotic medication and herbs. I cautioned her that non-pharmacological approaches take time and that she might not notice much of a change before our next appointment in 10 days. Since she was so depressed, I wanted to see her again soon in order to confirm that she was making progress.

Later that week she learned a kind of meditation called Transcendental Meditation. She also implemented some of the other lifestyle recommendations I suggested.

When she came back for her return visit, I told the medical student to first visit with Jane T. while I finished with my current patient. Ten minutes later I went to Jane's room and knocked on the door. I asked to speak with the medical student as I politely told Jane I would be with her in just a few more minutes. Outside the examination room, I asked the medical student for her impressions, and if she thought that anything had changed since Jane's first visit.

"I literally did not recognize her. I thought I was in the wrong room. Jane is smiling and making eye contact. It is really unbelievable," said the medical student.

As I met with Jane, she reported that she was no longer depressed, was sleeping better, and that her family life had markedly improved. She was already talking about wanting to go back to work part time.

The medical student, who had just witnessed how profound meditation can be was eager herself to learn this technique. It should be cautioned not every patient who learns Transcendental Meditation has such a rapid and dramatic response. Most Transcendental Meditation practitioners notice some improvement over time in some aspect of their lives.

The Importance of Meditation

The importance of meditation in this process of creating and maintaining health cannot be overemphasized. Meditation is not simply relaxation. It is the tool for developing higher states of consciousness and enabling you to become more aware. As your consciousness is expanded, you become sharply tuned in to your environment. Potential problems are foreseen before they even have an opportunity to manifest and are consequently avoided.

Meditation also purifies the nervous system, the mind, and the emotions. The profound rest achieved during meditation refreshes and rejuvenates the entire being. Consistent meditation therefore fosters a sense of balance that extends into all areas of one's life.

What is Meditation?

Meditation is a process by which conscious thought is transcended. This does not mean that you just stop thinking. Rather, the attention of the mind is turned away from the external world and back onto itself until all thoughts and impressions are let go. This letting go process has three key aspects.

First, the withdrawal of the concepts, perceptions, and thought patterns that consistently cloud our minds allows a break from their influence. This is particularly useful when emotional turmoil is present or when we wish to determine the function of the ingrained patterns of our thinking. The break that comes with this process of letting go allows you to return to your activities in the world with a clearer mind. You can then objectively decide to keep or discard these patterns of thinking once you have removed the judgmental part of your mind from your self as you do when in a state of meditation.

Second, the break the mind receives gives the nervous system a very deep and profound rest. This allows the stress on the nervous system to be released. When a deep impression is made on the mind, the stress is not easily erased. For instance, if you ever had the unfortunate experience of being in a car accident, the moment of impact and the adrenaline rush of the event imprint itself on your nervous system. It may become difficult to release the association you now have with a car, and you may even feel afraid every time you step into a vehicle. But through the deep rest in meditation, the nervous system is nourished and some of the stress of that experience becomes undone and lifted.

The stress-relieving effects of meditation take the relaxing quality of sleep one level deeper, as meditation allows you to delve beneath the surface of your feelings and thoughts and connect with that part of you that is always still and peaceful. Regardless of their size, stresses of all kinds can be ameliorated through consistent and deliberate meditation.

Third, when meditation involves transcendence, the source of thought is contacted. Pure consciousness or pure awareness is attained. This is the source of energy and intelligence that underlies all of the activities of the physical body. This is the source of healing, life, and liveliness and it is truly rejuvenating and regenerating.

Transcendental Meditation

The most effective meditation must involve the process of transcending. This is usually done with a tool that allows the mind to turn away from the external world and focus its gaze inward. This tool is called a mantra, a meaningless sound that has known impact on the nervous system. The most effective method for this process of transcendence is appropriately named, Transcendental Meditation.

Research on Transcendental Meditation has shown that the rest obtained during meditation is twice that of the deepest part of deep sleep. Oxygen consumption normally decreases about 8 percent in Stage IV sleep. In meditation it can decrease 18 percent or more.

This certainly has benefits in terms of nervous system function. It also has profound health benefits, because it provides contact with the source of health. It is not simply a break from stress or from life. Many studies suggest that meditation is more efficient at healing than sleep. The research findings document profound reduction in the incidence of disease. In some areas, such as heart disease, these reductions are as great as 92 percent.[4]

Not only are these findings indicative of healthier individuals but of lower health care costs as well. These significant improvements cannot simply be attributed to decreased stress. They are too large. Other dynamics in the health of these individuals must be involved. Beyond relaxation, this meditation provides increased awareness, real stress release, freedom from ingrained mental and emotional habits, contact with the inner source of energy, and intelligence that is the foundation for health.

While Transcendental Meditation is not the only form of meditation widely available in the United States, it appears to be the most efficient at providing these health benefits. It cannot be learned from a book; otherwise, instructions would be provided here. Transcendental Meditation is a technique that is taught one-on-one with a qualified instructor.

The Power to Heal

As you move forward in learning about your power to heal, pay attention to what you already know. In following the two suggestions of practicing meditation and allowing the body proper time to rest, you can potentially eliminate half of all the most common chronic diseases that affect Americans. By allowing the body proper rest and sleep, you can provide as much health as by consuming nutritious food.

Knowing and practicing these two methods of contacting the source of health provides you with great healing power. If you learn nothing else from this book, remember these two methods, and you have already within your grasp the ability to transform your life and your health.

4

REMOVING THE BLOCKS TO HEALING

The Drama of Ama

The concept of *Ama* is not part of Western medicine. Ama is a crucial part of the Ayurvedic understanding because it is what causes blockages in the flow of energy and intelligence. Ama is the buildup of toxins in the physiology that arise when we are unable to digest our food and/or process our life experiences productively. Ama blocks access to energy, liveliness, and intelligence. It leaves you feeling sluggish and heavy and can make awakening each morning feel very difficult.

Ama is described as:

- The consequence of poor digestion of food *or* experience.

- A toxin that builds up in the body and prevents our connecting to the body's underlying intelligence.

- Blockages — whether in our arteries, our eyesight, our joints, or our ability to experience love and happiness.

- Improperly digested food — any toxin or waste not utilizable by the body as food.

- Excess of any byproduct of metabolism that builds up in our bodies, such as uric acid, which can cause gout, or components of bile that can form gallstones.

- The products of maldigestion, which block the energy channels or Srotas of the body.

This concept is of such importance that it deserves a more thorough investigation. As we have discussed before, the body is more than a physical device. It is a conduit for consciousness. While the idea of energy or life force conveys some of the meaning, consciousness incorporates much more than just force. It involves intelligence, organizing ability, creativity and, above all, liveliness or bliss.

Consciousness is transformed and transmuted through the various layers of the human being — spiritual, mental, emotional, and physical. It is conducted from the largest switching stations in the body, the Chakras, through subtle and smaller channels all over the body. Consciousness is then delivered via these channels or meridians to all parts of the body.

When Ama blocks the flow on any level, pain or suffering is the result. Blockages by definition impede the flow of liveliness, intelligence, energy, and proper organization. They impede the flow of life itself.

The idea that pain is the consequence of blockage is very clearly represented when looking at a physical example. Take a tourniquet and place it on your upper leg. After a few minutes your leg will start to hurt. Lean your face on your hand long enough, and you get first numbness followed by pain, as the nerve flow is re-established.

If the outlet of a ureter is blocked by a kidney stone, you will get excruciating flank pain. Block the flow of the bile from the liver with a gallstone, and you get a stabbing pain in the middle of the back. Block the flow of an artery in the heart with a blood clot, and you get a crushing pressure in the chest. Block the flow of subtle energy in any muscle group, such as in the low back, and you get chronic pain. Even though we have clearly established that pain results from blockages on the physical level, what is not so apparent is how this also functions on other levels.

What happens when we block the normal flow of an emotion? What happens when we block the flow of desire? What happens when we block the tendency of the mind to go to a place of greater happiness or charm? What happens when the natural tendency to improve the mind is blocked? *Healing is blocked.* The natural flow of subtle life energy is blocked. And disease and suffering are the result.

In Ayurvedic medicine, the concept of Ama traces its origins to the beginning of Ayurveda when the system was first cognized, thousands of years before the American Medical Association began using the abbreviation AMA. Ama is created when food or experience is not fully metabolized. If digestion is not strong, then some part of the food or the experience is left unusable. These remnants then block the Srotas through which intelligence and energy flow in the body. These depositions may occur at any level of metabolism. Weak digestion, then, is the origin of the blocks to full functioning of the physiology. It is for this reason that digestion and its strength are considered just as important as food and the qualities that the food contains. One can eat the perfect food at the perfect time, but with weak digestion, the food cannot be metabolized, and Ama is the end result.

I often encounter patients overlooking the importance of digestion when undertaking various forms of nutritional therapy. They focus on what goes into the body, and not what gets utilized. They ingest massive doses of vitamins, but absorb very little of their content. This malabsorption is reflected in the individual's urine, which turns bright yellow as a result of the excess vitamins and minerals that are excreted from the organs.

We know from allopathic medicine that absorption varies widely from person to person. In some conditions, it is so poor it hinders treatment. A migraine headache is one example. When a person has a migraine, the stomach and intestines do not work normally. The normal peristalsis or movement that propels food along the digestive tract is hindered. Giving an oral medication to a patient with a severe attack of migraine simply does not work. This has spawned the use of injectable medications and intranasal medications that are absorbed through the fine blood vessels in the nose. Unfortunately, as is the case with this dangerous system of medicine, the injectable form of migraine medicine sometimes precipitates heart attacks. While a migraine is debilitating, its treatment is hardly worth the risk of a heart attack.

Taking large doses of vitamins does little if one is unable to absorb them. Furthermore, some nutritional programs actually hinder the body's ability to absorb and digest food. Many patients in my practice have tried an all-raw-foods diet. Others have greatly increased the amount of salad and other raw foods they consume.

While conceptually these approaches would seem to be healthy, the reality is that raw food is hard for the body to break down. It must be, in essence, "cooked" in the stomach. This is the only way to extract any nutritional value except fiber from raw foods. Not only are raw foods difficult to digest, but also over time they weaken digestion. In fact, they can weaken the digestive system so much that even cooked foods become difficult to absorb and metabolize.

Ama develops when food or an experience is not completely digested. Each time we eat on the run or rush right after a meal, digestion is hindered. In this setting, Ama will be created in all but those with the strongest digestive power. The classic Vedic texts give guidelines to encourage proper digestion and to prevent the creation of Ama. These guidelines can be organized in terms of improving digestion itself, picking and preparing foods that are better suited to complete digestion, and optimizing the environment for digestion and assimilation. I give my patients these guidelines:

IMPROVING DIGESTION
1. Eat when you are hungry.
2. Do not eat when you are not hungry.
3. Eat to only 75 percent full.
4. Do not eat until the previous meal is digested (3 - 6 hours).
5. Avoid large amounts of liquid before, after, or during meals.
6. Make lunch the large meal of the day.
7. Avoid ice-cold food and beverages.
8. Chew well.
9. Avoid large quantities of raw and uncooked food.
10. Do not eat when you are upset.
11. Do not eat too quickly or too slowly.

FOOD SELECTION & PREPARATION
1. Eat predominantly vegetarian food.
2. Eat organically produced food.
3. Avoid genetically engineered food.
4. Eat the freshest possible foods.
5. Avoid "sale" food that is old.
6. Do not eat burnt or rotting foods.
7. Avoid microwave ovens.

OPTIMIZING THE ENVIRONMENT

1. Eat in a settled, quiet atmosphere with a settled mind.
2. Do not work, read, or watch TV while eating.
3. Always sit to eat.
4. Eat at approximately the same times each day.
5. Take a few minutes to sit quietly after a meal before returning to activity.
6. Do not eat right before bed.
7. Consume food that is pleasant to both sight and palate.
8. Eat food that is prepared by a happy, settled cook.

When concepts such as the importance of digestion and the prevention of Ama are introduced, it is useful to have some guidelines. Who can live by such rules 100 percent of the time? I have yet to encounter anyone who can. If this is the case, do we simply go on accumulating Ama and becoming less and less vibrant and healthy? Realistically, that is what happens to many of us.

Even though many people attribute disability and the physical limitations that come with it to aging, Ayurveda instead reasons that the declining functioning of our health has more to do with the accumulation of Ama and the blockages in the appropriate transference of energy rather than by just age itself. As Ama collects, the physical system is blocked from recharging itself with vibrant energy. One area of the body after another seems to fail. A concrete example of a Srota that has Ama deposited in it is a clogged artery. Another example is when the blood supply to the tiny vessels of the brain is blocked, and cognitive function declines. Yet another instance is a joint becoming stiff and unyielding, as Ama prevents the flow of energy. And Ama deposited in the lens of the eye obscures vision, making cataract surgery a mandatory solution for treatment. All of these examples of age-related disabilities may sound dauntingly dismal, but the practice of Ayurveda offers hope to mitigate their effects and even, in some cases, prevent them from occurring.

The ancient physicians of India were responsible for tending to the country's royalty. One of their most important tasks was to ensure them long and youthful lives. With this understanding of Ama, they needed to not only prevent its accumulation, but remove it before it caused problems. They developed a science of purification that became a specialty in classical Ayurvedic training, much as rheumatology or dermatology is a specialty in allopathic medicine. This field is quite detailed in terms of its method and the substances used to eliminate Ama from the body. In brief, it centers on five therapies, each aimed at a different parts of the body and mind.

The name of this specialized training is *Panchakarma,* meaning "five actions." These represent the five basic purifications for eliminating Ama. The basic treatments are:

1. *Nasya,* or nasal administration of substances to purify the nasal and respiratory passages and the mental/emotional energies associated therewith;
2. *Vamana,* or therapeutic vomiting to purify the stomach and chest and the mental/emotional energies of those areas;

3. *Virechana,* or purgative administration to remove Ama from the small intestine and the digestive tract and to purify the subtle energies associated with these areas;
4. *Basti,* or enema therapy to cleanse the colon and the energies associated therewith;
5. *Raktamokshana,* or therapeutic bloodletting.

Each of these can conjure up disgusting images, but the process, when done properly, rejuvenates and refreshes the individual. It should be noted that bloodletting and therapeutic vomiting are no longer practiced and have been replaced by other more gentle methods of purification.

In recent years, newer and faster approaches to purification have been created to replace the traditional methods, which are by their nature, more involved and take longer. Naturopaths, for example, often emphasize colonics in which the colon is irrigated with water to clean out the toxins. Ayurvedic medicine regards this kind of purification as cleansing but also very drying to the intestinal tract and body. Just as getting in and out of the shower several times a day can leach the natural oils from the skin, so too can water enemas cause a subtle dryness. This actually drives imbalances deeper into the body tissues.

Ayurvedic Panchakarma methods require proper preparation of the body, specific selection and administration of substances, and an appropriate post-care routine. Ayurveda believes that without this kind of diligent supervision, digestion could actually be made worse by faulty administration of Panchakarma. The result would be enhanced

Ama accumulation in the body's tissues and imbalance in energy flow.

These days it is very common and almost fashionable for my patients to talk about doing a detoxification diet or program. Often this involves the unsupervised administration of herbs that have a laxative effect. Yet few realize the great potential for creating worse problems as they self-administer a do-it-at-home detoxification program.

Sarah's Story

Sarah H. had done a detoxification program. She came to me complaining of overwhelming fatigue and expressed a strong interest in doing another detoxification program. Even after our consultation, she followed through with her interest and self-administered a detoxification program involving strong laxative herbs. She returned to my office a few weeks later reporting insomnia in addition to other health problems.

Sarah is a classic example of someone who had good intentions to purify her body, but since she did not undertake the proper preparation measures, such as strengthening the body with herbs and ingesting certain oils to soften her, she further threw off the balance of her already delicate physique. This imbalance was consequently showing up as insomnia.

REMOVING THE BLOCKS TO HEALING

Proper Purification

Proper purification involves all levels of the human being — physical, emotional, mental, and spiritual. People often notice change on all these levels when undergoing Panchakarma therapy. Sometimes they are tempted to find meaning in the emotions and thoughts that come up in the process. But the individual should be forewarned that analyzing the thoughts and feelings that are triggered by the purification process has little value. If you liken these bubbling issues that surface during Panchakarma to garbage that has already been placed onto the curb for pickup, it is clear to see how this introspection is not encouraged in Ayurvedic medicine.

Purification is most successful when one is practicing meditation. Transcendental Meditation purifies and clears out those elements or vibrations induced by stress. Whenever experiences make a deep impression on the mind, stress is created. This happens whether the experience is a death in the family, an embarrassment at work, or even a wonderful surprise party. The pressure created by the impact of this experience alters the nervous system and impedes its future functioning.

The process of gaining deep rest in Transcendental Meditation allows the alterations in the nervous system to repair. The vibrations set up in consciousness are no longer reinforced. In this manner, consciousness is purified. The habit of transcendence purifies the deep impressions formed in the mind by powerful experiences. The mind becomes clearer and less cluttered. This process greatly aids the purification process of Panchakarma and makes it complete. From this level, the root of disease is ferreted out. Illness is prevented. Its story ceases, and the drama and havoc that Ama causes in the life are no more.

5

GETTING IN TUNE WITH OUR NATURE

The Doshas

Without proper balance, the physical system will eventually manifest a lack of coordination of intelligent functioning. This is a subtle process, which occurs long before the manifestation of disease. Our third imperative for health is that we must use our awareness to animate that which is life-giving and life-promoting for our individual nature. We must create balance and a lifestyle that puts us in tune with our true nature.

Doshas are thought to arise from the underlying field of energy and intelligence that Ayurveda understands is the basis for all life and creation. This precisely parallels what modern physics is discovering in its Unified Field theories. Physicists have realized Einstein's dream of unifying all the forces of nature in one grand theory that explains how all of creation comes from one Unified Field.

In describing the vibrations of the Unified Field, we can categorize them by their qualities or tones. The vibrations of music convey a certain feeling or mood. They can be dark and low or bright and airy. It is through this tone that the emotion of the music is communicated and feelings stimulated in the listener. In the same manner, the vibrations of the Unified Field can be classified by their tones. Through these tones, a style of functioning is imparted to the body. For example, one of the tones of the Unified Field is air-like. Just like airy music, it communicates lightness to the body. A little lightness is okay, but excess lightness causes wasting in the tissues and difficulty gaining weight.

The classically described tones of the Unified Field are:

- Space
- Air
- Fire
- Water
- Earth

These manifest in the body as pairs. The combination or Dosha of space and air qualities is called *Vata* in Ayurvedic medicine. The fire and water paired quality is called *Pitta* Dosha, and the water and earth quality is called *Kapha*

Dosha. It is through these Doshas that the manifestation of the body and its functioning are guided. The word *Dosha* means "impurity." This name is used because it is just a vibration of the Unified Field, a disturbance in the field, and not the pure essence of the field itself.

In order to remain in balance and prevent disease, the Doshas must be maintained in the proper balance. Being in balance is dependent on the individual constitution. Each individual has a different natural quality to the body. Some people are naturally stocky. Some people are naturally thin. Some people are naturally muscular. This natural physique is a manifestation of the underlying proportion of Vata, Pitta, and Kapha with which the individual was born. It is very important to understand that each individual has all three Doshas: Vata, Pitta, and Kapha, operating within him or her. It is rather a matter of degree as to what Doshas tend to have more or less dominance than the others.

A Vata person's constitution, for example, has more of the qualities of space and air. This gives him or her a more ethereal quality with a lighter and thinner physique. If this Vata person eats only an extremely light diet with foods such as raw vegetables and rice cakes as the mainstay, it will only create further imbalance. A slight individual eating foods that lack substance for long periods will aggravate the Vata element in the body, and health will not be maintained. The further into the Vata vibration the person goes, the further he or she will move away from wholeness.

63

As the individual accumulates more Vata, additional impurities will develop. This process of accumulation is a fundamental part of the creation of disease. The ancient seers who cognized the principles of Ayurvedic medicine described the series of steps in this process of imbalance. Six stages were described in all. The beauty of this organization is that by recognizing these stages, one can intervene early and rebalance the system, long before disease manifests. That is true prevention.

Vata Dosha

The basis of the three Doshas is a construction of the five elements: space, air, fire, water, and earth. Vata is a combination of the air and space principles, which are related to movement, and it therefore governs the bodily functions that control movement in our minds and bodies. The qualities of Vata are moving, dry, rough, light, quick, cold, coarse, and unstable.

Characteristics of a Vata Type

- Lighter, thinner build
- Performs activity quickly
- Tendency toward dry skin

- Aversion to cold weather

- Irregular hunger and digestion

- Quick to grasp new information; also quick to forget

- Tendency toward worry

- Tendency toward constipation

- Tendency toward light, interrupted sleep

- Speaks quickly, with irregular speech pattern

Even though any body type can have a Vata imbalance, a Vata individual will have a tendency to accumulate Vata more readily than other body types. Physical, behavioral, and environmental factors can influence this natural predisposition for a Vata imbalance by increasing or decreasing this Dosha to a point of imbalance.

Imbalanced Vata Signs

- Dry or rough skin

- Insomnia

- Constipation

- Common fatigue (nonspecific causes)

- Tension headaches

- Intolerance of cold

- Degenerative arthritis

- Underweight

- Anxiety, worry

An excess of Vata can also manifest as an emotional state of fearfulness, worry, insomnia, anxiety, loneliness, or emptiness. With too much Vata, pervasive anxiety, or feeling too "spaced out," frequently occurs. Physically, excessive Vata can be expressed as dryness, whether in the skin, nails, nose, colon, joints, or bones. Conditions are manifested in a variety of ways. For instance, in the colon, this dryness results in constipation. In the joints, the result can be osteoarthritis, which is the drying up of the synovial fluid that functions to lubricate the joints of our body. An imbalance of Vata is also associated with other conditions such as poor digestion, flatulence, sciatica, lightheadedness, dizziness and lack of coordination, or a general sense of not being grounded.

Since Vata is the Dosha of motion, and it influences the body's cycles and biorhythms, it is extremely important to be regular in lifestyle by establishing a daily routine in order to compensate for a relative lack of stability in the body's functioning. Thus, meditation and restful, deep sleep are crucial to achieve and maintain a balanced Vata Dosha. The following lists the qualities apparent when Vata is in balance:

Balanced Vata Signs

- Mental alertness
- Proper formation of body tissues
- Normal elimination
- Sound sleep
- Strong immunity
- Enthusiasm

If Vata is balanced, your internal clock will be regular and cyclic, and all changes and transitions within your physiology will be smooth. To pacify or calm Vata disturbances, three things are required: rest, regularity, and nurturance. Nurturance, from the Ayurvedic perspective, involves warm food, warm emotions as is found with emotional support, and physical warmth, especially with warm oil massages.

In order to balance Vata, consider the following:

1. Establish a daily routine, including keeping to a regular early bedtime no later than 10 P.M. Staying well-rested is essential for a balanced Vata.

2. Mealtimes should also be kept at the same time each day.

3. Vata types inherently need less vigorous exercise, so while physical activity is important, it should be of low intensity, such as walking, hiking, swimming, bicycling, or yoga.

4. Diet should consist mainly of warm, cooked, slightly oily, and wholesome foods at each meal. Eat fewer salads and raw vegetables, avoid all red meat, and reduce cold foods and drink, since these aggravate Vata Dosha.

5. Regular daily meditation is important for balancing Vata.

6. Daily self oil massage.

Abhyanga — The Ayurvedic Daily Massage

Abhyanga is the Ayurvedic oil massage. It is considered an integral part of the daily routine recommended by this healing system for overall health and well-being. Some of the benefits of this practice are enumerated in the traditional Ayurvedic texts: "It is nourishing, pacifies the doshas, relieves fatigue, provides stamina, pleasure and perfect sleep, enhances the complexion and the luster of the skin, promotes longevity and nourishes all parts of the body." Some of the other benefits classically describe include:

- Increased circulation, especially to nerve endings
- Toning of the muscles
- Calming for the nerves
- Lubrication of the joints
- Increased mental alertness
- Improved elimination of impurities from the body
- Softer, smoother skin
- Increased levels of stamina through the day
- Better, deeper sleep at night

The Ayurvedic massage is usually performed in the morning, before your bath or shower, to facilitate the release of toxins that may have accumulated during the previous night. It is sometimes prescribed for short periods of time before bedtime to treat sleep problems. Sesame oil is the traditional choice, although other oils may be recommended based on imbalance and body type by an Ayurvedic practitioner. Sesame is a very heating oil and for those who need more cooling effect, olive oil is often recommended. If you are using a pure oil that has not been herbalized, you may wish to purify or "cure" the oil. (See next page.)

How to Perform the Self-Massage

Massage oil should be warm. Store your massage oil in a plastic flip-top bottle and place it in the sink with hot water to warm the oil. Or place hot water in a large mug and place the plastic container in this. Squirt the oil into the palm of the hand and apply to the entire body, starting with the head first. Do not forget the ears, the scalp, or the feet. Also, at this time, if you are using pure unscented or non-herbalized oil, you can place approximately 2 tablespoons of oil in your mouth and hold it there, while swishing it between the teeth occasionally, as you do the rest of the massage. This practice is very beneficial for preventing gum disease.

It is best to place a large towel on the bathroom floor, so you don't have to worry about the oil dripping. After you have placed a liberal amount of oil on the skin of the entire body, massage the body, applying even pressure with the whole hand. Apply light pressure on sensitive areas such as the abdomen or the heart. Use more oil and spend more time where nerve endings are concentrated, such as the soles of the feet, palms of the hands and along the base of the fingernails. Circular motions over rounded areas, such as your head or joints, and straight strokes on straight areas, such as your arms and legs, work best. After you're done, allow the oil to soak in for 5 to 10 minutes. Do some other part of your daily hygiene routine at this time (shave or do nails or do some gentle yoga postures or just relax). Follow the massage with a warm bath or shower. Note: To get the oil out of the hair, place shampoo on the head before you put any water on. It will lather up a bit and save tremendously on the amount of shampoo you need to use.

To keep your pipes from clogging: Once a week put 1/4 cup of vinegar down the drain followed by 4 quarts of boiling hot water (from the stove, not from the faucet).

---

*Curing involves heating the oil. CAUTION: ALL OILS ARE HIGHLY FLAMMABLE. Use low heat, and never leave oil on heat unattended. To cure the oil heat it to 212 degrees Fahrenheit. If you do not have a thermometer, you can put a few drops of water in a pan with the oil — the water will sink to the bottom and start to boil and "pop" when the oil reaches 212 degrees. Remove from heat once this temperature is reached, cool, and store for use as needed. Cure up to a quart of oil at a time.

Precautions: Be careful not to slip in the shower, as oily feet are very slippery. Also, do not perform this self-massage if you have open sores or other skin issues or if you have sensitivity to oils like sesame or olive oil.

Pitta Dosha

Pitta is a combination of the fire and water principles and relates to heat and metabolism. Thus, Pitta governs bodily functions concerned with metabolism and energy production. The qualities of Pitta are hot, sharp, acidic, pungent, and slightly oily.

Characteristics of a Pitta Type

- Moderate build
- Performs activity with medium speed
- Aversion to hot weather
- Prefers cold food and drinks
- Sharp hunger and digestion; can't skip meals
- Medium time to grasp new information
- Medium memory
- Moles or freckles
- Good public speaker
- Tendency toward irritability and anger
- Enterprising and sharp in character

The most salient quality of Pitta is heat. Think of Pitta Dosha in the body as an internal combustion engine, burning food to keep your body's metabolism running. In physiological terms, Pitta Doshas represents bodily functions concerned with metabolism, particularly digestion.

Pitta is also responsible for metabolizing mental and emotional experiences. When Pitta is overheated, or out of balance, emotional experiences may include irritability, impatience, and a quick temper. Excessive hunger and thirst are characteristics of an imbalanced Pitta as well. So too, are skin rashes, inflammation of joints and tendons, and heartburn.

Imbalanced Pitta Signs

- Rashes, inflammatory skin conditions
- Ulcers, heartburn
- Vision problems
- Excessive body heat
- Premature graying or baldness
- Hostility, irritability
- Hot flashes
- Inflammation

In its healthy state, Pitta is decisive, efficient, well-spoken, passionate, and inspired by life. The following lists other qualities that are evident when Pitta is balanced.

Balanced Pitta Signs

- Normal heat and thirst mechanisms
- Strong digestion
- Sharp intellect
- Contentment
- Generosity

Therefore, when Pitta is balanced, digestion and metabolism will be strong, energy will be high, body weight will be perfect, complexion will be radiant, and cognition and emotions will be steady and positive.

Here are some tips to help restore Pitta to its unique and balanced state:

1. Pacify the nervous system by avoiding TV, computer, and the telephone after 9 P.M. Turn the lights out by 10 P.M. for a cooler and more restful night.

2. Pitta-type people tend to love competitive sports or goal-oriented activities such as bodybuilding or distance running. The most important thing for Pitta-dominant people to remember is not to strain and try too hard. They need to balance the heat in their physiology with cooling water and/or winter sports and yoga.

3. Ayurveda recommends a Pitta-pacifying diet emphasizing foods that are innately cooling to the body, such as greens, pomegranate, cilantro, lemon, and lime.

4. A Pitta-pacifying diet eliminates the unhealthy buildup of excess acids and other toxic by-products of metabo-

lism by promoting their elimination through the kidneys, liver, and bowel. Pitta-predominant individuals should eat organic, wholesome foods with lots of fresh vegetables and sweet, juicy fruits as well as spices with gentle diuretic effects, such as coriander and cilantro.

5. Avoid processed foods, junk foods, cheese, yogurt, red meat, hot spices, alcohol, caffeine, vinegar, sugary desserts, and fried foods.

6. Never skip or delay meals. Eat lunch by 12:30 P.M. and dinner by 7 P.M. To help cool the fiery quality of Pitta, be sure to drink plenty of fresh, pure water every day.

7. A soothing coconut oil massage every morning is excellent for Pitta types, particularly in the summer months.

Kapha Dosha

The Kapha Dosha is a combination of the earth and water principles, which represent the supporting structures and cohesion of the body. The qualities of Kapha are heavy, cold, slow, sticky, soft, oily, sweet, stable, solid, and dense. Kapha is responsible for strong bones, strong teeth, the capability of storing energy, and for immunity, strength, and stamina.

Characteristics of a Kapha Type

- Solid, heavier build
- Great strength and endurance
- Slow, methodical in activity
- Oily, smooth skin
- Slow digestion, mild hunger
- Tranquil, steady personality
- Slow to grasp new information, also slow to forget
- Slow to become excited or irritated
- Sleep is heavy and long
- Hair is plentiful, thick and wavy

In its less healthy or imbalanced state, Kapha manifests in the form of colds and flus, diabetes and obesity. Congestion is a sign of imbalanced Kapha. Congestion can take place on the physical and/or emotional level. An imbalance in Kapha can cause a congested personality and lead to complacency, being heavy-hearted, greedy, and lacking motivation. Lethargy is one of the main symptoms of Kapha imbalance.

Imbalanced Kapha

- Oily skin
- Slow digestion
- Sinus congestion
- Stiffness
- Fatigue
- Cysts and other growths
- Obesity

Kapha, in its healthy state, is strong, long-lived, calm, nurturing, forgiving, sweet-spoken, deliberate, and able to hold on to money and friends. Balanced Kapha gives a sense of being unflappable, stable, and profoundly loyal.

Balanced Kapha

- Muscular strength
- Vitality and stamina
- Strong immunity
- Affection, generosity, joyfulness, dignity
- Stability of mind
- Healthy, normal joints

Here are some helpful guidelines to help restore Kapha to its unique and balanced state:

1. Exercise. Since the morning hours of 6 A.M to 10 A.M. is Kapha time, it's important to avoid sluggishness by rising by 6 A.M. Exercise is a must for Kapha-type people since they are prone to obesity and are have motivation difficulties. Endurance sports such as rowing, distance running, and swimming are especially beneficial. Exercise to the point of working up a sweat is perfect for Kapha types but often too much for a Pitta- or Vata-type person.

2. Eat a light diet. Home-cooked meals complement the sensual and nourishing nature of Kapha types. Eat plenty of legumes, whole grains like barley and quinoa, and cooked vegetables. Spice generously with thyme, basil, mint, oregano, cumin, turmeric, fresh ginger, and black pepper.

3. Avoid red meat, dairy, cold drinks, and sugar.

4. Since Kapha types oily predispositions, oil massages are not required.

5. Stay motivated. The best thing a Kapha type can do to care for him or herself is to engage in moderate to strenuous physical activity 15-20 minutes each day.

Understanding Balance

The Doshas apply not only to body types, but also to every material object or item in creation. Thus, if you can describe a substance in terms of the Doshas, you can know its effect on the human physiology. Take a color, for example. The color blue is cooling in nature and will balance the fiery hot nature of Pitta. The sense of taste can also be used as an example. In examining salt, we know that salt's nature is hot since it burns right through ice. Therefore, it increases or aggravates Pitta and will throw it out of balance. On the other hand, it will offset the coldness of Vata and help to restore Vata's equilibrium.

In this manner by understanding our individual tendencies and our individual imbalances, we can design a program to stay in balance, one that puts us back in tune with our nature and re-establishes our contact with the Unified Field. In this process, we often must start with our imbalances first and then, later, follow a lifestyle that is appropriate for our doshic make-up.

Keeping your predominant Dosha balanced through lifestyle, self-care, and diet is fundamental to the prevention of illness according to Ayurvedic medicine. In the next chapter, we will explore not just the importance of prevention but its application according to Doshic type and how its practice works to restore the individual back to wholeness.

6

ULTIMATE PREVENTION

Heyam duhkham anagatam. (Avoid the misery which has not yet come.)

— Patanjali

Fundamentals of Prevention

The fundamentals of Ayurvedic prevention go far beyond early detection and far beyond the screening programs and yearly checkups of Western medicine. Once a year is hardly adequate to attend to the most important aspect of medicine namely, avoiding illness and the dangers it entails. True prevention is a daily practice, retuning and realigning oneself with one's nature and with nature itself.   As is the case with any discipline, the more attention spent on learning and comprehension, the more profound the result.

The way I characterize the essence of true prevention is derived from the three imperatives of healing. The actual steps to prevention are outlined below, followed by a discussion on how an individual can successfully address them.

First and foremost is re-establishing contact with the source of life, with the essence underlying any living system. Reconnecting with the underlying field of nature that nurtures, supports, and organizes the body is critical in this process of maintaining health and preventing disease. Opening one's awareness to this source of healing promotes healing in and of itself. By reconnecting with the underlying field of life that harbors the intelligence that structures the body, one re-establishes natural order within the body. Through repeated contact with the Unified Field, one naturally becomes more attuned with it, and harmony within the body is naturally maintained. Reconnecting with the source of life is the first fundamental of prevention.

The second principle in the ultimate system of prevention is purification. The process of purification is of prime importance. Without removing disharmonious frequencies or blocks to the proper flow of energy and intelligence in the body, life cannot be maintained in an orderly and vibrant manner. Without filtering out the impurities that block the flow of energy within the body, problems in the physical structure can only be managed, not resolved. Purification involves all levels of the human being: the physical, emotional, mental, and spiritual.

The third fundamental of true prevention is balance. After reconnecting with the source of health and purifying those blocks to maintaining energy and order, the system must be brought into proper balance. Each individual's body is different and requires different food, exercise, and routine in order for optimal functioning and health. One size does not fit all. The needs of a thin 5-foot-10-inch female and a heavy, stocky athletic 5-foot-10-inch male are vastly different. Rebalancing the system is necessary in order to maintain health.

Balance is necessary in order to prevent the development of blockages or damage to an area of physiological functioning. Often this aspect of Ayurvedic medicine is emphasized in other popular approaches, such as Traditional Chinese Medicine. Discovering one's body type and learning those things that are in tune with this type are given importance. However, this is only the third aspect of prevention. Without first reconnection and purification, balance will be an impossible juggling act because the root cause of illness and the essence of prevention will have been overlooked.

The fourth fundamental of true prevention is rejuvenation. Re-energizing and recreating the physical system requires nourishment. It requires nurturing on all levels, not just the physical level. Nourishment and nurturing are carried out through a dietary and nutritional approach that focuses on more than simple building blocks of amino acids and vitamins. Just as thoughts contain and project a certain vibrational energy, so too do those physical substances we call food. Two elements are important: the nature of the food or its qualities and the quality of vibration it carries, created from how it was raised, harvested, handled, and prepared. The ability of food to nourish and nurture is dependent on both. The essence of rejuvenation is contained in the energy that is transferred to the individual and the quality of this energy. Finally, general tonification (rejuvenation through the use of tonics) is a necessary part of this process, as purification and rebalancing require energy for their proper completion.

The fifth and most important fundamental of prevention is averting danger. Undertaking action in the present to avoid misery in the future is key to prevention. Yet, the means of averting danger is neither explicit nor fully developed in the allopathic approach to medicine. On a mundane level, this principle is expressed in certain actions, such as wearing seatbelts. Utilizing concepts from the consciousness model, we can see the potential for a more dynamic and impacting system of averting danger.

In the Unified Field, waves or vibrations are set in motion. The quality of these vibrations affects the manifestation process through which the physical body is created. Just as radio waves extend far beyond the radio itself, the Unified Field contains vibrations that come from quite distant space versus time events. It is through this field that we are connected with the rest of the universe, and it is through this field that other elements of consciousness or vibration affect us. These effects or influences are widely varied. They range from the effects of other people in our environment to the influences of others who are not in our immediate environment, but with whom we may have a resonating connection. They include everything from the collective vibration of society at a given time (also referred to as the collective consciousness), and to the vibrations produced by large bodies in space, such as planets and constellations.

Since the Unified Field deals with both space and time events, the vibrations we set forth in the past also echo back to us to impact our present situation. It is the understanding of these vibrations of the past, present, and future that gives rise to the body of knowledge called *Jyotish*. Through this knowledge, a sense of the trends of time can be gained and the possibility of prediction becomes possible. Knowing that the trend for a period of time may bring difficulties on the level of the body allows one to take action. By setting a different or counter-vibration in motion, one can cancel a damaging effect returning from the past or from some other energy in the universe. This is truly averting the danger not yet come.

Connection

If the source of life is the underlying field of consciousness that we contact daily, what need might there be for reconnecting with this? How does one become disconnected? Why isn't the infinite energy and intelligence contained within this field ever present in our experience?

While some connection with this field must be present for life to exist, the strength of this connection can vary. The extent to which we are in tune with all of nature and our own nature and act according to the dictates of the unique body we have been given determines the strength of our connection with the whole of life. If we set up vibrations that are out of tune with our nature, it will cloud and interfere with the energy and intelligence coming to us through the Unified Field.

How do we come to be out of tune with nature? Unlike cows, which do not eat pizza at midnight, we have been endowed with free will. Rather than having our intelligence ruled by the rhythms of nature, we have the capacity to use our intelligence in a free manner. We can ignore the dictates of nature and obscure our connection with it. In Ayurvedic medicine this is called the mistake of the intellect or *pragya-aparad*.

The intellect in this phrase does not have to do with being intellectual or liking books or anything like that. It refers to the finest thinking level where we are able to discriminate between this and that. It refers to our subtlest level of decision-making or discriminating between two options. It refers to our free will. We can choose to do something with an intellect no longer in tune with the underlying field of intelligence, and this leads to disharmony with nature. In other words, the fundamental mistake, which eventually leads to a disconnection from the Unified Field, is the mistake of an intellect that is not grounded firmly in the Unified Field.

Such an intellect is not directed by or in harmony with the underlying intelligence of nature. When we choose against our better judgment to stay up until midnight and eat pizza, our intellect has strayed from its source, and we go against our nature. Subtle though this may be, the constant repetition of acts and decisions out of tune with one's nature leads to the imbalance that creates disease.

Reconnecting with the Unified Field, with the underlying field of energy and intelligence, serves many functions. It recreates the flow of energy in the body. It re-establishes the organizing intelligence surrounding an area of the body. Finally, it grounds the intellect and allows it to become more in tune with one's nature, so that decisions are spontaneously correct and in tune with nature.

How does one reconnect with the source of life and re-establish the intellect in that field of intelligence? The answer is quite simple. Through deep rest, reconnection is attained. The deep rest of sleep and the deep rest that occurs with proper meditation restore the connection. As we have stated previously, the most direct and the most profound reconnection takes place with some select meditation techniques like Transcendental Meditation.

In this meditation, the mind settles down and opens to its source, the Unified Field, where connection is re-established. This process produces results on many levels, each adding to its efficacy as primary prevention. The intellect is re-established, and choices are made that are life supporting and life-enhancing. The flow of energy through the body is enhanced, and the intelligence organizing the body is put back into place, ensuring proper functioning.

Anna's Story

Anna came to me complaining of chronic fatigue. She felt her life was spiraling out of control. She was failing in her career and her relationships. She felt she could not function well because of her poor health. She did not have the energy to exercise and would push herself to do so, but then would end up with a cold or flu every three weeks. She felt her immune system was weak, so she took Echinacea on a daily basis. Because of her father's struggles with colon disease, she worried she would get ulcerative colitis, a condition in which the large intestine becomes inflamed, and the lining ulcerates and bleeds. She did have some symptoms of loose stool and felt something was wrong. Her family physician performed a battery of tests on her, and all of her results came back normal. She had a child who was just starting first grade, and although she was working only part time, she felt overwhelmed. She was looking for preventive medicine to avoid her father's condition, but she also wanted relief from her chronic fatigue. When I asked about sleeping habits, she said she was sleeping without problem. When I asked further, she stated she was going to bed at 11:30 and awaking at 6:30 to help get her husband off to work. She felt this was sufficient. I asked her how much she slept on the weekends. She said that she usually slept until 8 A.M. on Saturdays and was typically woken up by her daughter on these days. This gave me a clue.

I asked her to talk with her husband about taking care of his own breakfast for two weeks. I explained to her that in Ayurvedic medicine it was considered more natural to go to bed before 10 P.M. I requested that she do this and then sleep as late as she possibly could each day. I also requested that she learn Transcendental Meditation. I told her that in order to become truly healthy, she needed to recover from her longstanding loss of contact with the source of her energy. She did both.

When she came back in two weeks, she was a different person. No longer worried, she stated she felt human again. Her bowel problems were resolved, and she noticed that her sinuses were no longer congested, a problem she had failed to mention to me in our first meeting. Her sleep debt was so great she had slept 11 hours for the first three nights. Later, after she started meditating, her sleep requirements continued to decrease, and she was sleeping only eight hours. Curiously, she noticed that she no longer had a desire to stay up late at night. She spontaneously started going to bed even earlier than 10 P.M. because, as she explained, "I just feel better when I do that."

This is an example of reconnecting with the Unified Field through deep rest by attending to sleep and meditation. Her primary and secondary problems resolved, as the intelligence of each area of the body was re-established through its connection with the Unified Field. The energy that is necessary to maintain health and prevent disease is regained in the process. That energy necessary to live a full, happy life is found once again. Most importantly, this process of reconnecting with the source of life brings not only liveliness, but also intelligence. Naturally, one's choices are more life-enhancing and life-supporting. In Anna's case, this meant she "just felt better" when she began going to bed at an hour more in tune with nature.

While these elements of her new daily routine helped to eliminate her chronic fatigue and her bowel problem, the greater impact will come from having found the key to true prevention. With additional energy to meet the demands of her busy life, she will have less chance of falling ill. She will be making health-promoting choices spontaneously, without external prompting. As any physician knows, this is an ideal situation, where the individual spontaneously changes to a more health-promoting lifestyle.

Fortunately for Anna, reconnecting to nature was sufficient for her to heal. If she had had some blockage in the energy flow in the area of the bowel or the sinuses, she might have noticed some improvement in her symptoms, but not the complete resolution she experienced. While her symptoms improved, the real story is what she learned about prevention. Given her newfound health habits, she is at less risk for developing her father's ulcerative colitis.

Purification

In Ayurvedic medicine, purification is the key to blockages being removed from the body. Even though purification or Panchakarma was already explained, it is one of the fortes of Ayurvedic medicine because of its complexity and comprehensiveness. The process of purification is an involved one, because blockages can exist on many levels. Physical toxins, emotional barriers, and mental impasses all can serve to obstruct the full functioning of the physiology of the individual. When the body is burdened with blockages, the life force cannot transmit its energies down to the physical level. Disease, pain, and suffering are the result.

Balance

The third principle of prevention is balance. Without proper balance, the physical system will eventually manifest a lack of coordination of intelligent functioning. This is subtle and occurs long before the manifestation of disease. In order to remain in balance and prevent disease, the Doshas must be maintained in the proper balance.

A Vata person, for example, has more of the qualities of space and air in their constitution. They will tend to have a lighter physique and be smaller or thinner individuals. If, after purification, they eat an extremely light diet with foods such as raw vegetables and rice cakes as the mainstay, this will only serve to create further imbalance and problems. A light individual taking light foods for long periods aggravates the Vata element in the body, and health will not be maintained.

The further into the Vata vibration the person goes, the further he or she will be from wholeness. When more Vata accumulates, more impurity will be present. This process of accumulation is a fundamental part of the creation of disease. The ancient seers who cognized the principles of Ayurvedic medicine described the series of steps in this process of imbalancing. Six stages were described in all. The beauty of the system is that by recognizing these stages one can intervene early and rebalance the system, long before disease manifests. This is true prevention.

The stages in the creation of disease are described in Ayurvedic medicine as follows:

- Accumulation
- Aggravation
- Migration
- Relocation
- Manifestation
- Chronicity

Accumulation of the Dosha is the first stage in the creation of disease. So where does it accumulate? Each of the three Doshas exists in every cell of the body. Every cell needs energy and metabolism (Pitta). Every cell has a structure (Kapha). And every cell needs circulation to move substances in and out of it (Vata). However, there are natural places in the body where each of the Doshas resides in greater quantity. Vata, being composed of space and air, is located in greater quantity in those structures of the body that have a space-like or airy quality. Examples of these would be the colon and the urinary bladder. Pitta, having the fire quality, lives in areas where food is burned or where things are metabolized in the body such as the liver and small intestine. Kapha dwells in the chest and lubricates the joints. It is in these areas that Doshas accumulate when balance is not maintained.

The second step in disease manifestation is aggravation. As the vibration that creates the Vata Dosha accumulates, the Dosha intensifies to the point where it can barely be held in its natural seat. This intensification is called aggravation. Finally, when it can no longer be held in its natural place, it wanders forward. This is the third stage, called migration. Wherever weakness exists in the body, the Dosha tends to relocate. It starts to re-accumulate further but does so in the wrong place. If Vata leaves its seat and starts to reside in Pitta's seat of the small intestines, it then gives its qualities to the functions of Pitta.

Vata, being light, airy, and cold, brings these qualities to the metabolism that takes place under the rule of Pitta. In this manner, digestion starts to take on a light and cold quality, which creates problems of gas or air and indigestion because the cold quality of Vata does not have the heat to break down and metabolize the food. Eventually, some sort of malady will start to manifest which is the fifth stage in the creation of disease.

Finally, if the manifestation is simply managed and the underlying imbalance not attended to, the disease will become chronic. Adult onset diabetes is an example of a chronic disease that is usually managed but that can sometimes be reversed through Ayurvedic medicine. This is done by utilizing special herbs and diet, as well as altering the metabolism of sugar through purifying Ama out of the digestive tract and the fatty tissues of the body.

Balance is an important principle of prevention. Numerous books have been devoted to this topic alone and with increasing health-care costs, much more emphasis needs to be placed on preventing diseases rather than treating them. Prevention is a complicated subject because it must be based on the individual. One man's meat *is* another man's poison.

I often refer my patients to such books as *A Woman's Best Medicine* by Lonsdorf, Butler, and Brown or *Contemporary Ayurveda* by Sharma and Clark to get a more detailed understanding of their body type and how to keep it in balance. While conceptual learning is valuable, and the services of a physician trained in Ayurvedic medicine can be very useful in this regard, the ultimate knowing comes from inner awareness.

I emphasize to patients that guidelines are useful, but they are just guides, not rules. It is through developing one's intuition and one's awareness that one spontaneously knows what foods, routine, and behavior will be balancing for oneself. Again, meditation plays a significant role in prevention. Meditation expands one's awareness. Meditation develops one's intuition. Regular practice of meditation develops this inner knowing and allows balance to be easily gained and maintained.

Rejuvenation

After reconnecting with the source of life, purifying the entire being, and rebalancing the fundamental elements of the body's physiology, rejuvenation is required. Few people realize how much energy is lost during the purification process and the need for body to reclaim this lost energy.

There is a serious risk of adding to an already accumulating Dosha when rejuvenation is attempted without rebalancing the system. This will push the individual from the accumulation stage of disease manifestation to the next and most serious stage of aggravation. Fortunately, the science of purification expounded in Ayurvedic medicine is sophisticated enough not only to remove Ama, but also eliminate Dosha accumulations. This is why the preparatory steps and the post-purification steps are so essential to proper treatment.

Jody's Story

Jody L. came to me with the specific desire to restore her immune system. She had been diagnosed with a very early stage breast cancer, and after having this lump removed did not want to consider chemotherapy or radiation. She believed that the immune system was crucial to recognizing and destroying abnormal cells, and that by enhancing the immune system's function, she could prevent a recurrence of her cancer. Jody was also very fatigued. Prior to her diagnosis, she had been pushing herself to work full time and go to school. After finding out she had breast cancer, she stopped working and cut back on her school hours. It had been six months since her surgery, and her energy was still low.

Jody was taking a product containing bovine colostrum, Echinacea, astragalus root, and shitake mushroom to enhance her energy and immune system. She was also taking an Ephreda-based "herbal energizer," which helped her in the morning, but did not last until the afternoon. She noticed that if she missed this supplement in the morning, she was no better off than when she first started it two months prior. She wondered why she could not get her energy back. She worried that her immune system would not function without her supplements but recognized her current approach was not working well.

Jody and I first discussed how her Ephreda-based herb combination was most likely worsening her situation. Like whipping a dead horse, the stimulants in her herbal combination were only serving to make her more fatigued. Her already tired body was being charged in the morning but by evening, when the effects of the supplements wore off, she was drained. She could not make any gains in energy with this approach.

We also discussed the relationship between the immune system and Ama in the body and how the beautiful intricacies of the immune system cannot function in a coordinated manner when Ama is blocking the finer Srotas of the body. I recommended that she stop her supplements and immediately undertake Panchakarma treatments at The Raj, an Ayurvedic clinic in Fairfield, Iowa. After that, we planned to meet again for recommendations regarding her supplements. She was able to arrange a weeklong stay at The Raj shortly after our meeting and returned a month later to my office.

As with many of the other previous cases I've discussed, the entire office staff did not recognize her. She appeared 10 years younger. She was smiling and was conversing vibrantly. And, of course, my staff was wondering when they could go to The Raj for a week and experience the change that Jody had.

In reviewing the supplements Jody had been taking, I explained that it was now the appropriate time to begin taking some rejuvenating herbal preparations. I recommended an herbal formula called Amrit Kalash. The anti-oxidant properties of this formula have been researched extensively. Antioxidants are substances that eliminate from the body free radicals, or highly charged oxygen species that destroy DNA and other cellular functions. Many people take vitamin C and vitamin E for their antioxidant effects. Amrit Kalash was found to be 1,000 times more potent than vitamin C in scavenging free radicals in a study undertaken by Dr. Hari Sharma at Ohio State University.

Amrit Kalash is a fascinating combination of herbs. Not only is it a free radical scavenger, it also has two other interesting properties. First, it is a tonic that *gives* energy to the body, rather than whipping it to work harder at the expense of needed energy. It contains many potent tonic herbs described in the classic Vedic texts. Second, it improves digestion and assimilation so that one is better able to derive energy from one's food. This is as important as adding energy to the body. By addressing all aspects of digestion, Amrit Kalash prepares the way for rejuvenation.

It allows optimal use of the daily intake of food. It therefore serves as a double tonic, supplying restorative herbs while strengthening digestion in the process. It turns food into a tonic itself.

With this herbal combination and other Ayurvedic guidelines, Jody was able to regain her energy, her buoyant outlook, and has remained free of cancer since 2001. For Jody, rejuvenation required not only a change in diet and adding herbal supplements, but it also involved proper rest and recreation. Her health was enhanced by the deep rest of meditation and by proper sleep obtained at the proper time. For Jody, meditation has also become an integral and important part of her lifestyle. It helped her to maintain her energy levels and allowed her to return to work and school.

Rejuvenation is a fundamental part of prevention. Without sufficient energy, the channels collapse and become clogged more easily. The energy flow to a particularly weak area of the body cannot be maintained. Purification can eliminate some of the blockages in the area, but even the riverbed itself becomes a block if the stream dries up and its flow is too weak. Through rejuvenation, the functioning of the immune system is enhanced and true prevention is attained.

Averting Danger

The final and very pivotal component of prevention is averting danger. Unlike modern medicine, which waits until the disease has started to begin treatment, Ayurvedic medicine starts treating the individual long before disease has an opportunity to manifest. It accomplishes this task because the model on which it is based is not a purely physical one. Its methods for detecting imbalance prior to the manifestation of disease are many. The effects of a vibration accumulating in the energetic interface with the body are detectable events in Ayurvedic medicine.

This vibration affects the entire system, sends its vibration throughout the physiology, and is then felt by the trained physician. It affects the function of rhythmic events in the body, and these subtle vibrations can be detected in the pulse of the patient, long before a disease is present.

Pulse diagnosis is just one of several ways to detect vibrational effects. It is one of the most comprehensively described methods, and, given the right teachers, it can be systematically taught. The information in the pulse is quite extensive. To sit with an expert pulse diagnostician is sometimes unsettling as the trained fingers sense the subtle vibrations and messages. Untold aches and pains, discomforts and problems are communicated to the physician without words. One walks away wondering if all that can really be in the pulse or if the physician is psychic. Yet, when queried, the reply is definite, the vibrations are truly felt in the pulse.

Having regular pulse diagnosis is one way to avert danger and a beginning step to treat imbalances before they manifest as an illness. Pulse diagnosis is an ancient science that requires practice, but it is useful even to the unseasoned practitioner's hand. Even though it is only one of several ways of detecting imbalance, since the pulse is so central to life, it is often the preferred diagnostic method in Ayurvedic medicine.

Ayurvedic medicine recognizes the interconnectedness of all of life. In the consciousness model, human existence occurs on many levels. Each level of consciousness interacts with the next level, influencing it and exchanging information with it. When an emotional event such as anger takes place, the pulse speeds up and stress hormones are released. This is an example of the interaction between levels, namely the physical one and the emotional one.

On the higher energetic planes of life, effects are less local. Distant events and influences can impact the human being in subtle, yet discernible ways. The work of physicians such as Larry Dossey in exploring the impact of prayer on healing is an example of such distant effects. He and others have demonstrated conclusively the impact of prayer on outcomes in hospitalized patients. Praying for others does have an effect and obviously, it is not just through the physical level of life.

We are living in a sea of consciousness. When one of us creates a wave, it affects all of us. It is not just people who create waves. All of creation creates some sort of wave, depending on its level of consciousness. We exist in a body, yet the "real us" is a collection of energy and information that exists independently of the body and exists in this collective consciousness. In this manner, other aspects of creation serve as the home for other collections of consciousness. Their tone and influence creates waves in the sea of consciousness also. Very large bodies, such as planets, carry with them a very large collection of energy and information when viewed through knowledge of the Unified Field. The qualities of this consciousness also create large waves that affect us.

Understood from a purely physical model, the position of stars and planets can have almost no effect on our health. How could they? These bodies are far, far away. Seen from the consciousness model, however, these bodies are huge and carry with them a large consciousness whose tone and timbre can have a profound influence. The waves that are set up in the Unified Field are tidal waves compared with those of an individual human being. Knowledge of the tone of our local universe and how it will interact with the tone of an individual person is the previously mentioned field of study called *Jyotish*.

Understanding how these tones from our universe influence our earthly lives can help to predict impacts on the human body in the future.

This may seem implausible and confusing to some. If there is an attachment to the physical model and a lack of understanding of consciousness, then suggesting that large planetary bodies have an influence can seem farfetched.

Science has progressed faster than the common intellectual notion. Physicists are comfortable with nonphysical events, with virtual fields, and with action at a distance. But even many intellectuals are uneasy with the notion of planetary influences. Yet most hospital staff would agree that there is a difference in what happens at work during a full moon. They will acknowledge having to face more emergencies, more chaos, and more psychotic or psychological cases.

This science of the effects of consciousness emanating from a distance is the forte of Jyotish. The pure or true science is still being uncovered or rediscovered. It is sometimes referred to as Vedic Astrology. As this field of knowledge is made more and more complete, its ability to predict trends for a certain individual will become more and more profound. In terms of prevention, this creates the possibility of an ideal system, one in which events can be accurately predicted in advance.

Certainly, warning of a potential problem would be desirable. However, even with advance notice, the effects of some major events cannot be thwarted. One of the beauties of this knowledge of Jyotish is a field of study of what are called *Yagyas*. Through Yagyas, certain key vibrations are set up in the Unified Field to counter the influence of an oncoming wave. They can minimize its impact. As is known from physics, if you set up a wave at an identical frequency but different phase to an oncoming wave, the oncoming wave is cancelled out. In this manner, Yagyas can serve as a means to alter the events foreseen by Jyotish. Just as prayer was thought by most physicians 20 years ago to be useless in healing people, research on Yagyas will one day show their effectiveness in averting the danger not yet come. This has the power to become the epitome of true prevention.

Averting danger is the ultimate illustration of prevention. It ranges from the mundane level of wearing seatbelts to the subtle and sublime knowledge of cosmic events and how to influence them. In a culture so obsessed with immediate gratification and excess stimulation, preventing danger before it occurs is too frequently overlooked.

Many of us neglect to see the big picture as we go about our daily routines. We do not see the expanse of time and the influence our present actions have on the future. With meditation, though, broader awareness develops, and we are spontaneously drawn to actions that are life-supporting. Naturally, we develop behaviors that avert trouble for us in the future. With an expanded awareness, we are able to see the broad scope of life and know that the quality of our present action determines our future well-being.

"Avoiding the misery not yet come" is the ideal of prevention. With a new model for the human being, new possibilities are available to make this ideal a reality.

The Ultimate Prevention Program

Given these five fundamentals of prevention — connecting, purification, balance, rejuvenation, and averting danger — what would the ultimate prevention program look like? How are these principles put into practice? Here the crucial difference between the allopathic approach to prevention and the Ayurvedic medicine approach is apparent.

Ayurvedic medicine offers techniques and procedures that go far beyond admonishing patients to change their lifestyles or the early detection of disease. Ayurvedic medicine offers an understanding of how disease develops that incorporates all aspects of human existence.

The ultimate prevention program of Ayurvedic medicine is composed of several elements. The first is meditation, particularly Transcendental Meditation. This simple technique is a powerful health promoter and supports each of the fundamentals of prevention. It is no wonder that meditators require less than half the health-care resources of nonmeditators. The second element is regular Panchakarma. This should be done two to three times per year to ensure that purification is complete. The third element is education about daily routine and diet and how to balance the Vata, Pitta, and Kapha Doshas. Fourth, Amrit Kalash and other herbal tonics to strengthen and balance the system are often prescribed. Finally, periodic Jyotish consultations and appropriate Yagyas based on the Jyotish complete the program.

The goal of this prevention program is to safeguard against the majority of diseases and promote health and longevity. It will provide energy and enthusiasm for life and will be the future of medicine. It will assure enlightened health for everyone.

AYURVEDIC PREVENTION
MADE PRACTICAL

Ayurvedic prevention is not complex. In fact, it is common sense. It does require some guidance at first, as well as making prevention a priority. This chapter serves to detail some of the common-sense guidelines offered by Ayurvedic medicine. It serves to further explain some of the components of the prevention program recommended in this system of medicine. Moreover, it goes beyond the prevention program and addresses common concerns. The topics selected here are relevant to anyone interested in prevention, and they are important components of a healthy lifestyle. They range from diet and exercise to cancer and heart disease.

"Prevention is the strong suit of Ayurvedic medicine," one of my professors used to say. It contains detailed information about a wide variety of topics that hold relevance for modern life. Ayurvedic medicine holds the key for a science of prevention, so badly needed by the industrial nations of the world.

These topics help to further clarify some of the components of the Ayurvedic medicine approach to prevention. They address problem areas that I often encounter in my clinical practice. Their discussion draws on some of the classic Vedic texts and puts this knowledge into context. This knowledge has stood the test of time. Unlike atorvastatin, which is a cholesterol-lowering agent and has been on the market for less than 20 years, these Vedic principles have been utilized over thousands of years. Such understanding and experience in preventive health care is irreplaceable.

Some of the topics covered are common to the allopathic approach, such as diet and exercise. But with a deeper understanding of the human being, it will be evident that a more profoundly effective approach to prevention is present in Ayurvedic medicine. Other topics, such as meditation and sleep are not as commonly discussed in a modern discussion of preventive medicine. Nonetheless, these represent important topics in Ayurvedic medicine and will provide further insight into the comprehensiveness of this approach.

Meditation and Ayurveda

The importance of meditation in this process of creating and maintaining health cannot be overemphasized. If one examines all the fundamentals of prevention, one sees that each of them is enhanced by the practice of meditation. For this reason, any discussion of the Ayurvedic medicine approach to prevention must necessarily include a discussion of meditation in order to make it complete.

Examined from the view of prevention fundamentals, meditation addresses each one. It provides the most profound way of reconnecting with the source of life, the source of thought, and the source of energy underlying and pervading all of existence. It purifies the nervous system, the mind, and the emotions. Meditation is not simply relaxation. It is the tool for developing higher states of consciousness. It expands consciousness, allowing one to be more aware. Through this process of developing consciousness, one is naturally aware of the impact of lifestyle choices and behaviors on one's health and well-being. Balance is naturally enhanced through this practice.

The profound rest achieved during meditation refreshes and rejuvenates the entire being. Finally, with greater awareness, one is naturally more in tune with one's environment and consequently, one spontaneously averts danger. When one is in tune with nature, every aspect of the life is supported and upheld. In this manner, meditation serves as the most potent force in any armamentarium against disease.

Most people in the United States unfortunately misunderstand meditation. It is more than just a health technique or a relaxation technique. Meditation develops awareness. And all practices of meditation are not the same nor are they equally effective in developing awareness. Not all meditation leads to the same benefits or same goals at the same rate.

The misconceptions surrounding meditation are legion. The misconception that meditation is concentration is an example. This is mistaking the end for the means. Concentration is the result of meditation. Settling the mind is the means to it, not the other way around. When one reconnects with the most expanded field of consciousness, the Unified Field, then one's awareness is increased. Greater awareness brings with it a more settled mind and a greater ability to focus.

Similarly, another prevalent misconception is that meditation is relaxation. Because of this misconception, many people assume that any means of relaxation *is* meditation. Stress management courses and holistic health centers offer a hodge-podge of relaxation techniques under the guise of meditation instruction.

Popular mind-body experts, such as Herbert Benson offer the "Relaxation Response," as a unifying theory of meditation and claim that all meditations are the same. Scientific research on meditation has proven that all meditation is not the same. Relaxation is a by-product of meditation, not its essence. Relaxation is an effect of the process of meditation, not its purpose.

The purpose of meditation is the development of consciousness. Its goal is enlightenment. Enlightenment can be understood as a state where consciousness is so developed that all of creation is perceptible. All of reality is known on each of the planes of existence described in the consciousness model — emotional, mental, intuitive, and spiritual.

Enlightenment is a state of perfect attunement in which the individual's actions are spontaneously in tune with his or her environment. Enlightenment is experienced as bliss, 24 hours per day, as this is the ultimate reality underlying creation. In this state, terms such as non-attachment fail, for the equanimity that is gained comes not from self-restraint; but rather from the perception of a greater reality that brings with it the inner experience of happiness. When one's reality is that of poverty, every dollar lost or gained sways the emotions. When one's reality is that of the billionaire, a dollar here or there makes little difference.

With great inner wealth and with the great inner happiness that comes through a deeper and more profound experience and perception of reality, the description of nonattachment does not do justice to the daily life of an enlightened human. Developing enlightenment comes from experiencing the Unified Field deep within oneself. By transcending thought, this field is directly contacted and experienced. This is the purpose of meditation, to contact that underlying field of consciousness and thereby expand and develop the individual's consciousness.

As the process progresses, the individual becomes more aware, the mind becomes sharper, the body more relaxed. Spontaneously, one gravitates toward more life-supporting activities and habits that are more in tune with the environment. The feeling of being in the right place at the right time is the hallmark of the enlightened. All of their actions are spontaneously in tune with the environment around them.

The most profound meditation has as its side effect relaxation. But relaxing does not ensure that one is meditating or developing consciousness. The more profound the meditation, the more profound the relaxation.

Studies comparing Transcendental Meditation to Benson's Relaxation Response and Progressive Muscle Relaxation consistently show two things. First, the health benefits that accrue from the practice of Transcendental Meditation surpass those of relaxation techniques. A significantly greater decrease in blood pressure is observed. The decrease in health-care expenditures is greater. The length of life is longer.

Second, the practice of Transcendental Meditation is self-reinforcing because it contacts the source of life itself, which is blissful. Therefore, compared with these other techniques, the practice of Transcendental Meditation is pleasant and because it is enjoyable, it does not require discipline to maintain.

A further misconception is that one can learn effective meditation on one's own through selecting a *mantra* from a book. A *mantra* is a specific sound or meaningless word or vibration that is utilized in meditation. Many people are led to believe that one does not need a teacher to learn to meditate. After the detailed discussion of vibration in the earlier chapters, it is clear how faulty this reasoning must be.

One who is unaware of the effect of a vibration set forth in the Unified Field will have haphazard results when picking a mantra on their own. It will not be known whether this vibration is in tune with the individual and their nature, whether it is suitable for them or completely against their nature. Furthermore, in discussing the *amplitude* or strength of a wave, we saw that the power of a vibration or the energy gained by being in resonance with a vibration makes a significant difference in terms of the vibration's effect. So, picking a mantra from a book or trying mantras handed out without the guidance of an enlightened teacher is fraught with peril. One has no idea whether the vibration is what an individual requires or whether this vibration has any power behind it. A properly selected mantra creates a life-supporting influence and counters some of the less positive vibrations echoing back to an individual.

Another common misconception is that a mantra is not necessary in order to meditate. From my perspective, the ideal meditation technique has the following five qualities:

1. It carries the mind into direct contact with the Unified Field. It transcends thought to allow the mind to directly experience the source of thought and the source of life. When the mind is not completely turned back onto the Unified Field, some subtle or mystical experience or perception of the inner planes may be had, but the full power of the Unified Field will not be experienced. The most rapid development of consciousness will not take place unless even the subtlest aspects of the mind are transcended.

2. It is effortless and self-reinforcing. As the development of consciousness is not completed in a single sitting, the process takes time. The ideal meditation technique is one whose practice is self-reinforcing. It is pleasant and brings happiness to the mind and does not involve struggle.

3. It creates within the Unified Field a positive vibration that is in tune with the individual.

4. It utilizes a vibration in the Unified Field that counters destructive vibrations echoing back to an individual.

5. It utilizes a vibration that has large amplitude or that has great power behind it.

Without a mantra, one can try to force the mind to transcend, to go beyond thought. But this is very difficult. It is like trying to not think of an elephant. The more you do try, the more you fail. Not only is it difficult to transcend in this manner, but one also finds that the other aspects of an ideal meditation technique are lacking.

Regardless of whether an individual has been practicing Transcendental Mediation for many years or for two months, the results are quickly manifested. This is exactly what Robert Keith Wallace discovered when he studied the effects of meditation on brainwave coherency in people who had been practicing Transcendental Meditation for only a few months and found that they were as profound as Zen practitioners who had been meditating for 15 to 20 years.

Many meditation techniques are available in the United States today. Transcendental Meditation is one technique I know of that meets all five criteria of an ideal meditation. It is also a technique with copious research demonstrating its profound effects on health. For these reasons, this is the first technique I generally recommend for my patients.

In the history of medicine, the greatest advances in the overall well-being and health of the average person have come not through drugs or surgery. Public health measures have saved the most lives.

In the hospitals of yesteryear, long before the era of germ theory, infection and death rates were extremely high, particularly infant mortality rates. An astute physician developed an obscure theory that there was some invisible element that was being carried from patient to patient by the physicians and nurses in the hospital. He insisted that the staff wash their hands before touching each patient. Mortality dropped dramatically. With this public health effort, sanitation and sterilization became the norm, and as a result, thousands of lives were saved. Likewise, the biggest advances in the health of the average American today have come not through medical technology, but through life-style modifications like smoking cessation and dietary changes.

Let us hope that future historians will note that the next great advance in medicine of the 21st century is the wide-spread practice of meditation. Meditation has already been shown to do all of the following:[5]

1. Decrease hospitalizations by 55 percent
2. Decrease mortality in nursing-home patients
3. Decrease outpatient utilization of health-care services by more than 50 percent
4. Decrease blood pressure without drugs
5. Decrease cholesterol without drugs
6. Decrease cardiovascular disease 87 percent
7. Decrease suicides, homicides, and crime rate
8. Decrease recidivism rate in prisons

While Transcendental Meditation is not the only tech-nique available in Ayurvedic medicine, it is certainly the most important. It should be the first recommendation of any serious practitioner of medicine, because it unlocks the key to healing.

Nutrition

There is a tremendous amount of confusion on diet and nutrition in the United States today. Too much of the emphasis of modern nutrition is on the building-block theory of the body. This theory basically likens the essential nature of the body to a biochemical Tinkertoy set that has been constructed out of a variety of biochemical and mineral substances. If one simply supplies the appropriate building blocks, health is supposedly guaranteed.

We saw in the discussion at the beginning of this book that health is so much more than simply a physical phenomenon. The definition of health in Ayurvedic medicine is not physical at all. It is bliss or happiness. This cannot come from viewing nutrition as a matter of eating regularly and making sure that our food keeps within specific dietary fat and caloric limits. Certainly, the proper amount of food with appropriate mineral and vitamin content helps, but this barely scratches the surface of nutrition from the Ayurvedic medicine perspective.

According to Ayurveda, nutrition's purpose is to nurture. This nurturing takes place on each level of the human being, not just the physical. Food can convey intelligence, order, and energy. Food is just as essential to living an optimal life as reconnecting to the Unified Field is. This does not mean that food is just an energy fuel like gasoline. Food imparts its qualities to the eater. Food imparts its energy to the consumer. Food carries with it the consciousness of the cook.

To nurture an individual life is a formidable task. This undertaking goes far beyond putting calories in the mouth. Nurturing involves emotion and caring. It involves creating an atmosphere ideal for growth and well-being. Certainly, vitamins and minerals are necessary components for physical growth, but they are not the only components for nurturing.

Nutrition and nurturing occur on various levels. On the physical level, nutrition involves ensuring proper elements are present and avoiding known risks associated with a diet too high in fat or too low in fiber. On the emotional level, eating involves conveying a feeling of comfort, well-being and a sense of satisfaction and pleasure. When this is lacking, we sometimes have a tendency to overeat. We consume more and more food trying to nurture ourselves emotionally without satisfaction.

This is common in obese individuals or with individuals who have a binge-eating disorder. Even though they attempt to derive comfort from food, they eat in such a blinding and hurried manner they miss the opportunity to process the complete experience of eating. These individuals are starved for the nurturing aspect of food, not for its calories.

For those with these kinds of eating disorders, the food is often prepared without love or care. Fast food for instance, is not just empty calories, it is also devoid of nurturing energy. Additionally, when food is eaten so quickly the emotional satisfaction associated with tasting each bite is never realized. In this setting, overeating is perpetuated and obesity maintained. In non-obese people, the lack of nurturing energy within their food often manifests itself in some other form or problem such as chronic fatigue syndrome.

The final level of nurturing is on the level of consciousness. Food carries with it certain qualities that can be expressed in terms of the Doshas. Because these qualities affect the balance of the body, they have organizing power. They can be thought of as conveying information to the body that act like a key. They unlock and stimulate certain processes in the body that act to balance or imbalance the physiology. Food that is fresh, whole, and organic carries the full organizing power to the body. In that sense, it can be said to be "intelligent."

On a subtle level, food also acts as a conductor of vibration. The energy, emotion, and thoughts of the cook get intermixed with the intelligence and energy of the food and are transmitted to the eater. The consciousness of the cook plays a crucial role in conveying this energy. Often spiritual masters will pay particular attention to ensuring that the food they consume is prepared by their own cooks. They make sure this is the case for their pupils also. This is because they know that the consciousness of the cook is carried into the food and conveyed to those who eat it. If the consciousness of the cook is pure and the cook is happy and reverent, this will be passed on to those who eat the meal. If the cook is bored and frustrated, this too will be carried over to the level of consciousness to those who consume the prepared food.

In looking at prepared food in this manner, the soul of a bag of McDonald's french fries or a Wendy's Frosty is quickly called into question.

The most mundane level of nutrition is ensuring that the intake of minerals and nutrients is adequate. The next level of nutrition is ensuring the diet does not harm the individual. Avoiding excessive dietary fat and ensuring a proper amount of both vegetable and non-vegetable fiber is recommended. The third level of nutrition is recognizing the importance of nurturing the entire individual. The ultimate level of nutrition is recognizing food as medicine. How can food be considered medicinal?

In discussing the Doshas, we talked about the different vibratory qualities or energies that compose the body. Vata has the qualities of space and air and is light, changeable, moveable, subtle, cold, and dry. Pitta has the qualities of fire and is hot, burning, sharp, and pungent. Kapha has the qualities of earth and is heavy, moist, and solid. These qualities are present in varying degrees in each individual.

Each aspect of the body has different components of the Doshas normally at play at any given time. This intricate balance of the Doshas in the body can be influenced by many factors, food being a key one. As we have said, food has much more than just a biochemical value. It conveys its qualities to the body. For instance, light foods lighten the body, heavy foods make the body heavier, and dry foods dry out the body. Spicy, hot foods add flame to the body and in excess, inflame it. Cold foods cool the digestion and make the digestion run cold, so that it does not perform its functions effectively.

Most of us do not pay attention to these subtle but very present qualities of the food we eat. The next time you eat something, before you put it to your lips, think about its composition, where it came from, and the Doshic qualities it contains. With just this small awareness, you will likely see how what you are about to eat will resonate within your physical, mental, and spiritual body.

The qualities of food are more complex than just surface features like hot or cold, heavy or light, wet or dry. Bitterness, for example, contains dryness, coldness, and lightness. A bitter food such as chard or arugula imparts all of these qualities to the body.

The action of any substance, when understood completely in terms of its qualities, can predict its effects on the body. Bitter substances will cool the body, decreasing heat or inflammation in the body, decreasing moisture and mass, and making the body drier and lighter. Given this understanding of food, it can then be used in a medicinal way to treat or prevent certain illnesses and conditions.

Suppose we have a condition whose essence is hot and moist such as a pimple or small boil. A boil is an accumulation of moisture and substance — of pus. It is also an inflamed area of the body. Thus, it has both elements of Kapha with its earth-like and moist qualities and of Pitta with its inflamed qualities.

In allopathic medicine, boils or pimples are often treated with an antibiotic, such as tetracycline. Most antibiotics like tetracycline are intensely bitter, if one tastes them rather than just swallowing the pill whole. This quality is imparted to the body on all levels. Because it is a refined substance or a single chemical structure, the bitterness is extremely concentrated.

The effects on the body of tetracycline's bitterness can be understood in terms of its side effects, caused by its intensity. In 10 percent of people, tetracycline causes gastrointestinal irritation, resulting in nausea, vomiting, loss of appetite, flatulence, diarrhea, or dry mouth. Since bitterness has a drying effect, the dry mouth side effect is easily understood.

The stomach protects itself from the acid it uses to digest food with mucus. Mucus is a Kapha substance. Since bitter decreases Kapha, it will cut through the mucus in the stomach and decrease its amount. Thus, the stomach's mucus lining will be disturbed and the stomach will be exposed to acid. Tetracycline's known side effects of nausea, vomiting, loss of appetite, flatulence, or diarrhea can therefore be explained within this dynamic interplay between the body's and the drug's qualities.

Tetracycline can also suppress bone growth because bitter is also catabolic, thereby consuming its structure and making the bone lighter. Other side effects are light-headedness and dizziness. According to Ayurvedic principles, bitterness creates lightness in the body and in its functioning. The list of tetracycline's side effects is very long, but the most common ones can be understood from knowing the underlying qualities of its taste. The challenge now becomes how to impart the benefits of a drug like tetracycline without also causing its uncomfortable side effects.

On a continuum of medicinal substances, herbs are less potent than antibiotics, but they also induce fewer side effects. Goldenseal is a very bitter herb that is considered to have antibiotic, antibacterial, and antiseptic properties. It is prescribed in various forms in herbal medicine for inflammatory and infectious conditions.

Since it is bitter in nature, its use can easily be surmised. Goldenseal's bitter quality should not be used by people with vertigo, who are emaciated or who are chronically debilitated. As stated previously, bitterness produces lightness and can therefore result in light-headedness to someone who is already prone to faintish qualities such as a person with vertigo. It can also further deplete or lighten an individual who is already wasted. Yet, it is not as fraught with side effects as is tetracycline, because it is not as purely bitter. It is buffered by the other substances within the plant. However, it must usually be taken longer than tetracycline in order to have an effect, as its onset of action is also much longer.

Further along the continuum of medicinal substances that can be used to treat conditions are spices. For those who want to or need to avoid the side effects of herbs, spices can alternatively be used. They are much better tolerated than antibiotics or bitter herbs. Bitter spices could be used to gently convey this same effect to the body. Again, the effect is less immediate and requires a longer period of administration, but its benefit is present nonetheless. Coriander is an example of a bitter spice that is often used to treat a variety of ailments.

Finally, at the extreme end of the spectrum, bitter foods can convey the qualities of lightness and dryness to the body. They too can have anti-inflammatory effects. But the duration of administration is much longer, often months before the effects are noticed. One of the advantages with using food as medicine is that it has almost no side effects.

Food can also be used preventively. Before a boil erupts, the excess Kapha and Pitta in the body can be detected by an experienced Ayurvedic medicine physician. Prescribing the right food and spices can rebalance Pitta and Kapha and prevent the boil from ever developing.

Herein lies a vast field of study in the art of prevention. The effects of foods on the body and their utilization as medicine is a detailed and comprehensive discipline. By using foods to rebalance the body before disease arises, food becomes much more than just sustenance and nurturance. It becomes preventive medicine.

The ancient Ayurvedic physicians recommended that diet consisted of the following: *Fresh food, freshly prepared by a pure and spiritual cook, consisting of an essentially lactovegetarian diet, adjusted to one's body type, one's imbalances, and the season of the year.*

This means preparation and selection of food are as important as the type of food. As we have already discussed, food is a vehicle for conveying energies influential qualities and subtle effects. Adjusting these to the individual and to their particular needs is a precise and thoughtful form of cooking that is not widely practiced in our culture. Our concept of a gourmet chef is one who can make extremely complex and tasty rich foods. The Ayurvedic concept of a chef is a true expert in the art of cooking that is as adept at creating health as is a physician. The cook then cultivates the exact influence that is needed by an individual and delivers it in as potent a form as possible. Reviving this art will make this kind of a chef a revered professional in the future.

Numerous findings from modern research support the Ayurvedic recommendation for a lactovegetarian diet and verifies the ancient seers' suggestion. I often tell my patients that if I could get all of them to do these two things — meditate and eat a vegetarian diet — I would save more lives than if I spent every day of my life only writing prescriptions.

Eating a vegetarian diet has been shown to have many health advantages. Cardiovascular risk with a vegetarian diet is much lower. Vegetarians have fewer heart attacks, less coronary artery disease, and less chance of developing congestive heart failure. They also have a lower cancer risk for many types of colon cancer, such as colorectal cancers. In addition, they have less gallbladder disease, less kidney disease, and much lower rates of diabetes. I recall that during my medical residency a man with severe coronary artery disease was discharged from the hospital. His cardiologist recognized the role of diet in his condition. He told the patient, "If the rabbit doesn't eat it, you shouldn't eat it either."

The reductions in cancer are dependent on the type of cancer, but for cardiovascular disease, the decrease is for all conditions associated with heart-related maladies, such as strokes and heart attacks.

Dr. Dean Ornish is widely known for recommending a low-fat vegetarian diet to his patients with coronary artery disease. Reductions in the risk of disease by 30 to 90 percent are unheard of even with most medical interventions. However, this one intervention of eating a vegetarian diet can bring with it great reduction in the risk of disease. Fortunately, this simple lifestyle change affords these wonderful benefits without reliance on drugs.

If one examines the gastrointestinal tract of carnivores versus herbivores, one finds that the structure of meat-eating animals is very different from vegetarian animals. The small intestine of meat-eaters is short and their teeth, which are designed for cutting, grinding, and chewing, are sharper than those of herbivores. They also have fewer molars.

The human being's physical characteristics more closely resemble the structure of an herbivore's.

As humans we tend to be very fond of animals even though our treatment of animals raised for food in this country is fraught with ethical and sanitary problems. One must wonder then if before consuming a hamburger, we had to slaughter it ourselves, would the rate of vegetarianism increase? Few people know that slaughterhouses have the highest employee turnover rate of any job, and slaughterhouse workers often suffer from depression and nightmares.

There are many misconceptions about vegetarianism. For example, there is a myth that protein deficiency is a danger with a vegetarian diet. If one is getting adequate calories, it is extremely difficult to become protein deficient on a diet with any sort of variety. Most foods, including grains and legumes have a large enough percentage of their calories from protein to easily sustain a human being.

Moreover, few people know that the Recommended Daily Allowance (RDA) of protein exceeds the actual requirements of a healthy human being. The protein recommendation was based on an average male weighing 175 pounds. Consequently this recommendation is an overestimate for the average female who weighs approximately 150 pounds. In order to be sure to meet everyone's protein needs, a 30 percent "fudge factor" for the average male was added, increasing the overall requirement by 30 percent. Hence, the actual requirement is far below the RDA for most individuals.

Studies have shown that only 8 to 12 percent of all caloric intake needs to be from protein in order for healthy survival. It is impossible to eat a diet that has any variety at all without getting at least this much protein. In other words, if you are eating enough calories to sustain your weight, you are getting enough protein. The exception to this would be if the calories you consume were coming from a single food such as brown rice, or an extremely limited diet such as brown rice and salad. Many weight-lifters and body-builders have successfully gained strength and muscle mass on vegetarian diets.

The myth of protein deficiency is furthered inadvertently by one of the proponents of the early vegetarian movement, Frances Moore Lappé. She wrote in her first book, *Diet for a Small Planet*, that vegetable protein was incomplete and that food combining was important in order to get the right amount of usable protein. Unfortunately, the chicken egg had been taken as the standard for the complete protein. Studies now show that it's not necessary to couple foods together in one meal to create a complete protein. Rather, your body will still manufacture a complete protein if you eat rice in one meal and a legume in the next.

Lappé, in later editions of her book, downplayed the complete protein requirements and started expounding the virtues of vegetable protein. She switched the focus of her vegetarian recommendations to a varied diet, and she de-emphasized the need for food combining.

Unlike the mid-1980s, when vegetarianism was still considered a fad, today, most people in the U.S. have now been exposed to someone who has adopted this lifestyle. They know firsthand that people do survive well without meat. Many people attracted to Ayurvedic medicine already are vegetarian or are leaning that way.

On the other hand, the use of milk in Ayurvedic nutrition is often under scrutiny. Many see milk as the cause of various health problems and assume that they are lactose intolerant. Milk is regarded as one of the best foods in all of Ayurvedic nutrition. It is praised as pure and wholesome — a tonic without equal. Why is it thought to be so beneficial, and why is it implicated in so many digestive problems in adults in the United States?

Recall that from the perspective of Ayurvedic medicine the energy of a food is as important as its nutrient value. This energy is derived not only from the qualities of the food, but also from how it is raised, the consciousness of those who raise it, and the manner in which the food is obtained. If the money to purchase the food was obtained through life-supporting and life-enhancing means, it will carry this energy to the body. If the money was obtained through impure means, such as profits from a cigarette company or from gambling, then the energy of the food will not be as life-supporting. From the perspective of Ayurvedic medicine, no food is equal to milk in terms of its purity as long as it is produced from cows raised in a benevolent manner and as long as the cows are being fed a diet of grain with no added antibiotics or growth hormones. No other food in nature is produced without loss of life. No other food is given freely for the nurturing of another being.

Most of the problems with milk come from two facts: People do not know how to prepare it, and their digestion has been weakened through many years of poor eating habits. Milk is a meal in itself and should usually be consumed after boiling it with spices to make it easily digestible. Boiling relaxes the protein structure of the milk, just as frying an egg alters the structure of the white of an egg, making it opaque. When milk is consumed in this manner and combined with a proper diet and eating habits, most people are able to digest milk and milk products.

Milk has many beneficial properties for the lining of the gastrointestinal tract. Those who consume milk products are less likely to develop colon cancer.[6] A recent study showed that women who take milk regularly were half as likely to develop breast cancer.[7]

Given this understanding, the Ayurvedic recommendation of a lactovegetarian diet makes sense. In this light, let us re-examine the recommendation of Ayurvedic medicine:

Fresh food, freshly prepared by a pure and spiritual cook, con-sisting of an essentially lactovegetarian diet, adjusted to one's body type, one's imbalances, and the season of the year.

Fresh food is considered important because food loses its energy the longer it is kept. Even in a refrigerator, the energy of the food is not maintained for long. Almost everyone can detect the difference between fresh-squeezed orange juice and orange juice from a carton. Attempts to genetically alter food so that it lasts longer are deceptive. Even though the engineered food can be transported over greater distances and will have a longer shelf life, it will have no value in terms of its life energy. Life energy, or *Prana*, is what is important in terms of real nourishment.

Genetically engineered foods should therefore be avoided. They may contain identical quantities of vitamins and minerals, but they do not nourish. It is a veritable abomi-nation that the regulatory agencies in this country do not require labeling of genetically engineered foods. While many do not choose to be sensitive to the energy of their food, those who are should at least have a choice in select-ing nongenetically engineered foods. Until the labels on food become more stringent, eating organic foods is the only guaranteed alternative to avoid consuming these other substances.

The Ayurvedic principle of only eating fresh food is in con-trast to the "Tuesday is leftover night" policy that many households adhere to. According to Ayurveda, leftovers do not have the vibrant energy of freshly prepared foods. The longer a food is left over, the less Prana it contains. The refrigerator, while convenient, may be simultaneously robbing us of our energy and health. This is not to say that everyone should get rid of his or her refrigerator. But chronically eating leftovers and frozen foods leads to both energy depletion and Ama accumulation over time.

Few of us have had the opportunity to experience nutrition in the Ayurvedic manner by having meals prepared for us by a spiritual cook who uses food as a means to recalibrate our physiology. Lacking this experience, we have become habituated to a less than ideal way of cooking and eating. But by being introduced to this style of eating, one is forever cognizant of the contrast between real nutrition and empty calories.

Recreation and Exercise

In keeping with the quantitative nature of modern medicine, exercise is often viewed in terms of calories burned, oxygen consumption or oxygen reserve, or cardiac reserve. Maximal and optimal heart rate measures are used by exercise physiologists and trainers to determine the impact a type of exercise has on the exerciser's health. In our culture, exercise is literally a workout where if there is no output of pain, no benefits are gained. Quantitative exercise is typically not recreational. We do it to stay fit, get our heart rate up, and build muscle. And most of us get a confidence boost too after a workout.

Exercise in the perspective of Ayurvedic medicine is intended to be restorative rather than exertive. It is intended to recreate the flow and connection of energy in the body and aid in the body's regenerative process. Recreation is to re-create. By reconnecting with the natural flow of energy, exercise re-establishes the renewal process that takes place with the daily turnover of cells in the body. This process of re-creation is greatest when the exercise focuses on flow in the body. It is furthered by movement that is subtle rather than fatiguing. Moreover, it is enhanced by the enjoyment of movement and the feeling of refreshment that comes when the energies of the body flow smoothly and properly throughout the body.

The ideal exercise from the Ayurvedic perspective is what is commonly called yoga. By its Sanksrit definition, yoga means "union." Yoga is really a science of union with the Unified Field. Hatha Yoga is that branch of knowledge that involves reestablishing flow through the Srotas and reconnecting the flow with its source through postures.

Too often the emphasis in yoga is on the posture and the exact position of each part of the body within that posture and not on its subtler aspects. Often advertisements feature photographs of the impossibly twisted positions achieved by someone whose flexibility looks more catlike than human. Yoga, when practiced for recreation and health, is an art that can be done by even the most inflexible. Young and old can practice it. Its emphasis is on awareness of the body and enhancing the flow of energy through awareness, not through torture or painful over-stretching.

Yoga is the ideal form of exercise from the Ayurvedic per-spective, as each posture allows the awareness to be focused on critical paths in the body. This awareness is like water to a plant. It provides nourishment and returns liveliness to that area. It refreshes as it rejuvenates. Yoga is true rec-reation because it recreates.

Also valued in the Ayurvedic perspective on exercise is walking. Walking is good for anyone of any age. It con-nects you to nature and is a great antidote to clearing a con-fused mind.

Different times of day are prescribed for different imbal-ances. Walking in the moonlight is said to be very good for cooling off the fire element of Pitta. Walking in the morn-ing is stimulating and helps to counter the sluggishness of Kapha that is present at that time of day and it is much kinder to the fragile joints of Vata types.

Physical training, regardless of its nature, should be gentle and gradual. Few individuals are suited to run a marathon or be a triathlete. Unfortunately, it is often the very thin individual who gets addicted to running and turns up with joint problems years later. Thin people have a great deal more of the space and air elements in their joints, which are characteristic of those with a dominant Vata Dosha.

Movement aggravates Vata and therefore increases other qualities of Vata, such as dryness. The joint space of the overly active Vata individual dries out, and the joint begins to become hardened with osteoarthritis. This is an example of exercise that is undertaken out of harmony with one's nature. While jogging may be good for Kapha types, it is not good for everyone.

Adjusting the type of exercise to benefit the individual is an important part of the Ayurvedic prescription in terms of lifestyle and routine. However, yoga and walking are considered good for all types, unless a specific injury or deformity is involved. Yoga reunites one with the source of life in its ultimate form. It recreates and regenerates the body. It is the epitome of exercise. It is true recreation.

Daily Routine

As already noted, the time of day alters the effects of exercise. We are part of nature, and almost every aspect of our physiologic functioning is affected by the cycles of the sun, moon, and planets. The sun's influence and the effects of light and darkness are particularly powerful.

The cycles of hormone release and their regulation of the body's functioning are related to cycles of light and darkness. Sunlight has direct effects according to one's location and the time of year. The absence of sunlight has been associated with depression. Many people in northern climates with little midwinter sunlight suffer from seasonal affective disorder (SAD).

From the perspective of Ayurvedic medicine, different times of day have different qualities. Kapha time, from 6 to 10 A.M., is the time of day when the dew lies on the grass, when the heaviness of morning makes for slow and lethargic movement. It has the qualities of Kapha, being moist, heavy, and slow. From 10 A.M. to 2 P.M. is Pitta time, when the sun is brightest overhead and the fire element is strongest. Vata time is from 2 to 6 P.M., when light, active qualities are greatest. The cycle then repeats itself through the evening and night hours.

Each of these times promotes certain activities. For example, Pitta time, being full of fire, is good for digestion and metabolism. Having the large meal of the day at noontime is recommended in Ayurvedic medicine. This is more in tune with nature and with human nature.

Many people suffer from reflux and heartburn and esophageal diseases such as ulceration and a transformation called Barrett's esophagus. Many sufferers could be spared these problems by knowing and adhering to this meal-timing recommendation. Often people with gastroesophageal reflux disease (GERD) are helped greatly by this simple alteration in lifestyle. They have been in the habit of eating their large meal at night, as do most Americans. Thus, they have little time to digest their meal before going to bed.

Lying down when stomach acid is still processing the meal causes its contents to be forced up against the esophagus, and the stomach acid burns. While the normal processing time, or transit time through the stomach, is approximately two hours, when digestion is out of sync with normal body rhythms, the transit time can be up to six hours.

Not all reflux disease is cured or prevented by switching the large meal of the day to noontime. Often other imbalances must be addressed in order to cure this condition. Even so, a large percentage of GERD is handled easily with this simple recommendation. It costs nothing. Its side effects are better health and better digestion. Each year billions of dollars are spent on this condition, which could be avoided with just this small capsule of Ayurvedic health education.

Not only is the cost of medication and testing enormous, but GERD is not always benign. Esophageal ulcers, which result from GERD, can bleed and sometimes result in death. Furthermore, constant irritation of the esophagus causes cells in this area to transform, resulting in the so-called Barrett's esophagus, a precursor of esophageal cancer. Barrett's esophagus is monitored very closely because it is known to transform into one of the deadliest of cancers.

The knowledge encompassed by this ancient wisdom of Ayurvedic medicine is simple and inexpensive, yet it can form the basis for preventing many conditions and can save many lives. This example of eating the main meal of the day at noontime, when Pitta is highest and digestion is best, is only one area where this is so.

135

When Vata is highest during the midafternoon, the mind is light, moveable, and creative. This is a great time to tackle new projects or solve a word puzzle. Understanding the concepts of the qualities of time allows one to organize the rest of the day according to optimal energies.

Those who have a tendency to become drowsy after lunch will protest that afternoon is the worst time for mental activity. Generally, sluggishness after a meal is a sign that digestion is weak and that one has eaten too much for the digestion to handle. The body has to utilize all of its energies to process the food, as the intake has been too heavy and too great for the body to handle easily. Also, those who are chronically sleep-deprived will sometimes notice sleepiness after consuming a large meal.

Food satisfies and relaxes, so if sleep has been cut short, the body will try to recover whenever the person relaxes. Furthermore, the full effect of a particular time of day does not come on like a switch. Pitta time does not last until 1:59 and then at 2:00 suddenly become Vata time. The transition is gradual. Therefore, the greatest effect in terms of Vata time will be experienced at the midpoint of the cycle around 4 P.M.

Some activities, by their nature, tend to aggravate the Doshas or throw a particular element further out of balance. To prevent this, activities are undertaken in a particular time that will balance out the activity. Vigorous exercise, for example, is inherently Vata-aggravating. Movement and motion, by their nature, aggravate the quality of Vata. Vata is light and quick and has the quality of the wind, which is fast-moving. Vata is responsible for movement in the body, for the flow through the channels, and for the body's movements such as peristalsis or movement along the digestion tract. By exercising in the middle of Vata time, one is increasing movement (a Vata quality) at a time when Vata is already dominant. This results in further unbalancing.

Exercising in Pitta time also is not ideal. It not only harms digestion, it unbalances Pitta. Exercising over lunch, in order to fit this important element of lifestyle into the workday, injures digestion. It suppresses normal hunger and metabolism. If vigorous, exercise not only aggravates Vata, but also heats the body. Adding heat at noon — in the middle of Pitta time, when the fire element is the greatest — aggravates Pitta.

The ideal time to exercise is Kapha time. Kapha's qualities are opposite to Vata's qualities in almost every aspect. Because Kapha time is heavy, moist, and sluggish, it balances out the Vata qualities of exercise, such as quickness, lightness, and dryness (one gets thirsty exercising). Since the cycles repeat themselves, some mistakenly attempt to exercise in Kapha time at night. This is the time when the body is settling down for sleep. Exercising at this time wakes the body up. It raises the body's core temperature and throws the natural cycle of body temperature off. It should be noted that core temperature naturally drops at night. Exercising at night wakes one up and can cause insomnia in those with Doshas already out of balance.

Therefore, Kapha time in the morning is best for exercising.

In this manner, the ideal time for each element of the daily routine can be organized. The most important activities have already been discussed — having lunch be the main meal of the day and exercising in Kapha time. The ideal routine from the perspective of Ayurvedic medicine is as follows:

1. *Arise by 6 A.M.:* Waking up in Vata time is ideal. Vata gives the qualities of lightness and clarity to the mind. Awakening past 6 o'clock gets further into Kapha time and makes it difficult to awaken. One feels sluggish and groggy. If one can get to bed early enough to awaken before 6 o'clock naturally, that is ideal. Following the full Ayurvedic routine and being in bed before 10 o'clock ensures that this occurs naturally.

2. *Evacuate the bowels:* Waking stimulates the digestive tract to start moving. This, coupled with the change in position from lying to standing, creates a natural downward movement that stimulates the urge to defecate. This is considered the ideal time to have a bowel movement. Sitting on the toilet for a few minutes and sipping some warm water to further increase peristalsis helps the process of elimination.

3. *Exercise:* A brisk morning walk or doing a long set of yoga postures or even both is ideal exercise for everyone. Communing with nature and reconnecting with one's environment are natural therapies for restoring and maintaining balance in life. For those involved in more vigorous training, exercising without stressing or straining the body is ideal. For most individuals, this means

keeping the maximal heart rate below 135 beats per minute. If the resting heart rate, taken first thing in the morning before arising, jumps more than five beats per minute, the exercise from the previous day was too vigorous.

4. *Oil Massage:* Abhyanga, or daily oil massage, is considered an important part of the daily routine in Ayurvedic medicine. The only exception to this would be an individual who has accumulated Ama excessively. Oil massage is said to calm Vata and prevent the multitude of diseases created by unbalancing Vata. The *Charaka Samhita* says the following in regard to daily oil massage:

Of one whose head is every day saturated with oil, headaches never appear, nor baldness, nor the effects of decrepitude; the hair of such a man does not fall off. The head and skull in particular, of such a man acquires great strength. By anointing one's head with oil one's senses become clear, and the skin of one's face becomes good; one gets sleep easily, and one feels ease in every respect.

By applying oil every day to one's ears, one becomes free from all disorder of the ear born of Vata, wry-neck, lock-jaw, hardness of hearing and deafness. As an earthen jar if saturated with oil, or a piece of leather if rubbed therewith, or the axle of a car or cart from application of the same substance, becomes strong and capable of resisting wear and tear, even so, by application of oil, the body becomes strong, the skin improves, and all disorders due to Vata are dispelled.

Through such means the body also becomes capable of enduring exercise and fatigue. Vata is chiefly instru-

mental in the sense of touch. The sense of touch has the skin for its refuge. For the skin, the application of oil is highly beneficial.

Hence, one should daily anoint the skin with oil. A person, by using oil every day, acquires smoothness and fullness of limbs, strength and beauty of form. When overtaken by old age, slight symptoms only appear.[8]

Self-massage with oil is not part of our culture. It seems foreign to us. More and more, though, people in the U.S. are beginning to recognize the benefits of massage therapy. Increasingly, Americans are going to massage therapists and many therapists use oil as a way to lubricate the skin and knead the muscles and joints.

5. *Oral Hygiene:* While the oil from the self-massage is sinking in, oral hygiene can be attended to. First, observe the tongue for a thick white coating, which is evidence of Ama or having eaten food the day prior that was too heavy or rich. Next, scrape the tongue with a tongue scraper or toothbrush. Floss and brush the teeth. Then, sesame oil should be taken in the mouth and used as a gargle or rinse. The teeth and gums should be rinsed in the oil and the oil swished through the teeth. The oil should then be held in the mouth for about five minutes. During this time one can shave or clip nails or attend to other hygiene matters.

6. *Shower:* A warm shower should be used to cleanse the body and remove most of the excess oil that has not soaked into the body. It is also recommended that one use a gentle glycerin soap and leave a little of the oil on the skin to protect it from getting dried out. Regular soap is too drying to the skin and can damage it. Wash-

ing one's hair is easiest if one puts shampoo on the oily hair directly before putting water on it. It will lather even without water, thus conserving shampoo otherwise, one has to shampoo the hair several times.

7. *Meditation:* Early morning is an ideal time for meditation. Although rising before Kapha time starts (6 A.M.) is recommended, it is ideal if one can naturally arise early enough to exercise and shower and still have time to meditate in Vata time. Vata gives clarity to the mind and gives a more profound meditation. This is a subtle point and not worth cutting sleep for. However, if one gets to bed well before 10 o'clock, one should arise in time to meditate before 6 o'clock naturally. This is the ideal.

8. *Breakfast:* A light breakfast according to the needs of the body, season, and imbalances is important. Few people should skip breakfast altogether. Doing so will tend to make one eat a larger evening meal than is healthy.

9. *Work:* Purposeful work that does not strain one mentally or physically is the ideal recommendation from the Ayurvedic perspective.

10. *Lunch:* The main meal of the day should be at noon. One should take sufficient time away from work to have a hearty meal. Attempting to take lunch in 20 minutes is much too hurried. Sitting for five to 10 minutes after the meal aids digestion. This should be followed by a very brief walk, a hundred steps or so according to some experts in Ayurvedic medicine.

11. *Work:* Late afternoon would be the best time for intense mental work. It is the time of day when the mind is clearest for mental activity.

12. *Meditation:* Meditation before dinner is ideal for several reasons. Attempting to meditate after eating is counter-productive, as the body is busy increasing metabolism to digest the food, rather than settling for the meditation. During meditation, the body settles and digestion is halted. Furthermore, meditating late at night can cause one to be refreshed and have too much energy to fall asleep easily.

13. *Dinner:* Dinner should be light. It should be what most Americans consume as breakfast, in terms of proportion and foods.

14. *Relaxing/Socializing:* Evening is not a good time for working or for stimulating entertainment, such as movies. These excite the mind and can cause difficulty with sleeping. Evening is best for relaxing or mundane activities and for pleasant socializing. These types of activities allow the mind to relax and let go of the day's events.

15. *Sleep by 10 P.M.:* One takes advantage of the heaviness and sluggishness of Kapha time in order to make falling asleep easy. This means one should prepare oneself for sleep and be in bed *before* 10 o'clock in order to be asleep by 10. If it takes one 20 minutes to fall asleep and 15 minutes to get ready for bed, then one should start the process at 9:25 P.M. at the latest.

This is the daily routine that is recommended from an Ayurvedic perspective. Each of the aspects of the routine is organized to maintain ideal health. Each has its rationale. Medical science will hopefully document this in the future. For example, the use of sesame oil in oral hygiene has great preventive effects on gum disease. Gum disease often disappears merely by following this simple procedure. The Ayurvedic routine is an important part of prevention in Ayurvedic medicine. It is not costly, nor is it complicated. One must only make the time and effort. One must only recognize the importance of small steps in treading the path towards health and longevity.

Longevity

In Shirley MacLaine's book *Out on a Limb*, she describes learning a breathing technique as part of her meditation practice. In explaining this technique, her instructor tells her that breath and life are intimately intertwined. He tells her that if she learns to control the breath, she can control life. He uses an example: giant turtles breathe about four times per minute and live to be more than 200 years old. When her instructor asks her if she wants to be 200 years old, she says she does not. When she asks him if he wants to live to be 200, he says, "No, I just want to go home." This story points out some of the myths surrounding longevity that are ingrained in us.

Living a long life is associated with being decrepit. Old age is thought to be a time of debility and fragility. We associate it with a lack of function and an inability to care for oneself. Our concept of old age often represents our fears. In this common view of old age as decrepitude, who would want to live to 200 years old?

As the section on daily oil massage suggests, the Ayurvedic thinking is quite different. Even this one simple act of oil massage is said to ward off decrepitude, rendering it without significant symptoms:

"When overtaken by old age, only slight symptoms appear."

The reality of old age in the U.S. is far from our common conceptions. The vast majority of elderly never end up in a nursing home. The majority do not lose their mental faculties. Increasingly the elderly are an active, involved group, both politically and personally.

The Shirley MacLaine story also points out another assumption: Aging is considered inevitable. No one would want to live to 200 years old if it entailed a hundred years of decrepitude. Aging is not inevitable in the view of Ayurvedic medicine. As the body replaces each cell, or the component of each cell, it is capable of "remembering" the blueprint for each one and for the organization of the cells as a whole. This replacement process need not, in and of itself, become inefficient or altered. Aging is not a requirement.

In the ancient descriptions of Ayurvedic medicine, a purification procedure for restoring youth exists. The procedure takes place over several weeks and requires living in seclusion, while the process is administered. During this time, the hair may fall out, teeth may loosen, but when the process is complete, a 70-year-old person is said to look 30 years old again. The knowledge of this procedure has been obscured and, because it is so drastic, it requires an expert physician to perform it. Tradition says that this procedure is done only periodically — every 50 years or so.

To most people, this seems like fantasy. Their concept is that aging is inevitable and cannot be reversed. Evidence to the contrary comes from studies on people who practice Transcendental Meditation. When typical indices of aging, such as blood pressure, near-point vision, hearing acuity, etc. are tracked for meditators, they are found to age much less. Typically, someone who has been practicing Transcendental Meditation for five years has a biological age 12 years younger than his or her actual chronological age. Several studies have been published on this reversal of aging.

What are the limits of reversing aging? The full force of the entire knowledge of Ayurvedic medicine has not been brought to bear on this subject. No one has studied aging in those who undergo Panchakarma or purification techniques. The most profound techniques of Ayurvedic medicine to reverse aging have not been brought out yet.

Certainly, we know of cultures where it is not uncommon to live to 115 years of age. How far can this be pushed with the ancient knowledge of longevity? *Ayurveda* actually means "truth of life" or "knowledge of longevity." What secrets might it hold for extending a productive and happy life far beyond what is commonly thought to be a normal life span? If one views the process of regeneration of the body, one cannot help but think in terms of immortality, or at least in terms of approaching immortality.

Shirley MacLaine's story also points to immortality. Her instructor's comment about just wanting to go home means going back to the source of life and living in that enlightened state. From this perspective, experiencing the non-changing, ever-present nature of the source of life *is* experiencing one's immortal nature. Immortality of the physical body can only be an expression of the experience of the immortal nature of one's consciousness. "Going home" means returning to this underlying field of consciousness, experiencing it, and identifying with it. In this way, immortality is experienced on the nonphysical level.

Our concept of aging often determines how quickly we age. Those who think young do live longer. It is frequently when one's purpose in life is lost, or when one feels that one's time is up, that death comes quickly. Anyone in the health-care profession has witnessed this phenomenon: An elderly person just wants to live long enough to see a beloved grandchild marry; soon after the event, the grandparent passes away. What is not appreciated is that thought carries with it energy, and this energy communicates and resonates with the body. The body is influenced by and responds to this type of thinking. While it is not the only determining factor, it does make a difference. Aging may be more of a self-fulfilling prophecy than a necessity.

Following the daily routine of Ayurvedic medicine — practicing meditation, practicing yoga, and undergoing seasonal purification routines of Panchakarma — all serve to rejuvenate the body and maintain youthfulness. The limits of this science in promoting longevity are unknown.

Conclusion:

The Power to Heal is in You

The Power

Without having to study modern medicine, you now know the basis for healing. Through the ancient wisdom of Ayurveda, you have the means to regain, maintain, and improve your health. This wonderful science of life is still being rediscovered. Its secrets have yet to be revealed in all their glory. Still, the truth of life has been rediscovered and through the knowledge of Ayurveda has become accessible to each and every one of us. That truth is that the power to heal is in you.

Ayurveda is knowledge worth knowing. It is a study that will serve you again and again. It is a field as vast as all cre-

AYURVEDA — THE POWER TO HEAL

ation, because its subject is the wholeness of all creation, whether it be an ecosystem, an elephant, or a human being. Understanding the role of consciousness, of your awareness in the process of health is the secret behind Ayurvedic medicine.

This book is only an introduction to Ayurveda. It is impossible to detail in these few pages the complex and vast knowledge it contains. The essence of Ayurveda is a message of hope: You contain within your being all that you will ever need to recognize any imbalance, any dis-ease and to heal it.

You have more control over your health than a legion of medical specialists. With the knowledge of Ayurveda, you have the ability to take charge of your destiny and prevent even the most serious disease. It is the only real health insurance available to you. Taking control of your health not only empowers you but it affects all those with whom you have contact.

Ayurveda offers you the means to tap into the greatest power any human can ever possess — the power to make one whole again. It is my hope that this introduction to Ayurveda will inspire you to learn more and to incorporate this knowledge into your life. With this knowledge we can hope for a day when disease and suffering will be a thing of the past. For the beauty of Ayurveda is its simplicity. It is something that can easily be passed from friend to friend from generation to generation and from culture to culture.

It is my hope that you will take the power to heal and spread it everywhere.

Blessings,
Paul Dugliss
November 25, 2006

References

[1] A. Chandra Kaviratna and P. Sharma, *Charaka Samhita* (Delhi, India: Sri Satguru Publications), 160.

[2] *Ibid.*

[3] William C. Dement, *The Promise Of Sleep* (New York: Delacorte Press, 1999), 263.

[4] Orme-Johnson, David, *Psychosomatic Medicine*, Sep-Oct; 49(5):1987, 493-507.

[5] See Roger Chalmers, Geoffrey Clements, Harmut Schenkluhn, Michael Weinless, Eds., *Scientific Research on the Transcendental Meditation and TM-Sidhi Programme, Collected Papers* (Netherlands: MVU Press, 1989).

[6] Jarvinen, P. Knekt, T. Hakulinen, and A. Aromaa, "Prospective study on milk products, calcium and cancers of the colon and rectum," *European Journal of Clinical Nutrition* 2001 Nov;55(11):1000-7.

[7] A. Hjartaker, P. Laake, and E. Lund, "Childhood and Adult Milk Consumption and Risk of Premenopausal Breast Cancer in a Cohort of 48,844 Women — the Norwegian Women and Cancer Study," *International Journal of Cancer* 2001;93:888-893.

[8] A. Chandra Kaviratna and P. Sharma, *Charaka Samhita* (Delhi, India: Sri Satguru Publications), 46-47.

[9] Shirley MacLaine, *Out on a Limb* (New York: Simon and Schuster, 1983)